R. C. CURRAN

COLOUR ATLAS OF
HISTOPATHOLOGY

Colour Atlas
of Histopathology

BY R·C·CURRAN

MD · FRCP (Lond.) · FRC Path. · FRS (Edin.)
PROFESSOR OF PATHOLOGY, UNIVERSITY OF BIRMINGHAM
AND HONORARY CONSULTANT
TO THE UNITED BIRMINGHAM HOSPITALS

FOREWORD BY SIR ROY CAMERON FRS

WITH 765 PHOTOMICROGRAPHS

HARVEY MILLER ~ OXFORD UNIVERSITY PRESS

ORIGINATING PUBLISHER: HARVEY MILLER, 20 MARRYAT ROAD, LONDON SW 19 5BD, ENGLAND

© 1966, 1972 R · C · CURRAN

FIRST PUBLISHED 1966

REPRINTED WITH MINOR REVISIONS 1967, 1968, 1969, 1970

REVISED EDITION 1972

REPRINTED 1973, 1975 (TWICE), 1976, 1977, 1978, 1979, 1981, 1982, 1983

Published in conjunction with OXFORD UNIVERSITY PRESS
Walton Street · Oxford OX2 6DP

Oxford · London · Glasgow
New York · Toronto · Melbourne · Wellington
Kuala Lumpur · Singapore · Hong Kong · Tokyo
Delhi · Bombay · Calcutta · Madras · Karachi
Nairobi · Dar es Salaam · Cape Town

Published in the United States by
OXFORD UNIVERSITY PRESS · NEW YORK

ISBN 019-921002-0

MADE IN SWITZERLAND

LITHOS BY SCHWITTER AG · BASLE

PRINTED AND BOUND BY ARTS GRAPHIQUES COOP SUISSE · BASLE

CONTENTS

FOREWORD by Sir Roy Cameron, FRS

HISTOLOGY is the keystone of pathology. On it are built our precise knowledge of how man's tissues behave when caught up in disease and the devices by which the signs of disease are derived from distorted function of tissue cells. Histology also goes a long way in explaining how the agents of disease are spread through the entire organism or eliminated by natural methods of defence. There is no corner of medical science into which it does not penetrate.

Nowhere is this role of histology better displayed than in the historical development of pathology. Many centuries of naked-eye recording of the ravages of disease, and of searching for reasons why men die, reached a turning point when the genius of Morgagni transformed the descriptive anatomy of disease into a science. By shifting the emphasis from the dead to the living, the aches, the pains, the distorted appearance and behaviour of the sufferer could now be viewed against a tapestry of abnormal structure. But this was not enough since these organs and tissues could, in turn, be unravelled, first into membranes and fibres, and later, with the advent of the microscope, into cells and their derivatives. The youthful Virchow, familiar with the discoveries of the biologists Schleiden and Schwann, saw clearly a new theory of disease based upon perverted cellular function and structure. By incredible industry and clear thinking, he steered pathology past its next landmark. Half a century of vigorous technical improvement in the preparation of tissues for closer and closer examination, aided by the introduction of aniline dyes, by Carl Weigert and the young Ehrlich, for the display of cellular components completed the evolution of our science. The modern era has witnessed the harvesting of a crop of discoveries and the perfection of techniques based on chemistry, optics and the like, whose outcome we can scarcely imagine at the present time.

Some of these contributions, so clearly derived from the histological approach to disease, are well worth recalling, for they should reconcile the over-worked medical student for the long hours spent at the microscope. Barely an hour goes by in the diagnostic practice of a busy hospital or an up-to-date practitioner, a public health laboratory or a medical research institute, in which the microscope is not used with skill and understanding. And microscopic anatomy not only helps greatly in finding out why a patient is ill and the likely cause of his condition but it traces, with great accuracy, the course and the progress of the disease, the response of the patient to treatment, the day-by-day changes in the disease pattern. Likewise it brings to light such living agents as bacteria, viruses and parasites, which initiate so much human suffering; indeed, it may arouse suspicion of an unsuspected agent or of a toxic substance in the cell territories and so intensify the investigator's attack on what seemed an insoluble problem. In the diagnosis and assessment of the spread, complications and outcome of tumours, and in the recognition of pitfalls that confuse them with less sinister conditions, histology plays a supreme part. No one can deny the need for proper training in a discipline so vital to the making of an efficient, well-balanced doctor.

The atlas so expertly and lovingly prepared by Professor R.C.Curran is a vivid reminder of all the arguments I have listed in the preceding paragraphs. It does not pretend to cover the whole realm of special pathology; that, indeed, would require a series of monographs prepared by many experts, and could have no place in the training of medical students and young pathologists. The devoted care with which Professor Curran has selected his preparations, aided by his masterly concise descriptions, and by the splendid colour photography that reproduces so faithfully the actual sections, places teachers and students alike under no mean debt to the author. May his book meet with the success that it so surely deserves.

November, 1965

PREFACE to the revised edition

Since it first appeared in 1966 the Atlas has been well received throughout the World, and has been published in four languages. Opportunity has been taken of the numerous reprints to correct errors and up-date the text. The reception accorded to the volume suggests that the selection of illustrations was generally satisfactory, and in this new edition the changes have been confined to those fields where significant advances have taken place, as, for example, in glomerulo-nephritis, or where insufficient attention appeared to have been given in the first edition, as in wound healing. The changes, which it is hoped will add to the value of the book, have been made without any increase in its size.

I should like to take this opportunity to thank Dr. C. W. Taylor and Professors D. B. Brewer, W. Thomas Smith and D. H. Wright for the advice which they generously gave during the revision of the text and to Dr. P. A. Judd for help with proof reading.

April, 1972   R.C.C.

INTRODUCTION

At a time when an over-full curriculum presses heavily on them, students welcome adequate instruction in histopathology. They are quick to appreciate the fact that only through knowledge of the alterations in fine structure that are demonstrable in most diseases can they understand how the disordered function characteristic of disease is produced.

The illustrations in this Atlas are from my personal collection, which is in current use for the instruction of under-graduates, and the book has been planned with the needs of this group in mind. At the same time it is hoped that the Atlas will prove of interest and value to postgraduate students training in the various branches of medicine and particularly in pathology. The lesions illustrated are, with a few exceptions, common or fairly common conditions, likely to be encountered in any large teaching hospital within a reasonable period of time. All the photographs are in colour, since in my experience students have considerable difficulty in recognising under the microscope the features shown in black-and-white photomicrographs. Special stains have been avoided, except for a few instances in which they are needed to make clear the essential feature of the lesion, and ordinarily haematoxylin- and eosin-stained sections have been photographed. Magnifications have not been quoted, since I believe them to be of little value, partly because processing of tissues for sectioning inevitably changes cell sizes in haphazard fashion, and partly because a cytological 'yardstick' in the form of lymphocytes or red cells has been included in as many pictures as possible. However, smears of peripheral blood and marrow form an exception, and with these comparison of cell sizes is essential. With most of them the same magnification ($1050\times$) has been used.

The text has been kept short in order that the essential histological features can be quickly assimilated and in the expectation that the student will at the same time read a full description of the disease in one of the many excellent textbooks of pathology that are available. The Index, on the other hand, has been made as comprehensive as possible; the names of lesions and also component parts of the illustrations, such as the many different cell types and special histological features, have been included to make easier the task of locating a lesion or a particular histological change.

I am deeply grateful to a number of colleagues for help in the preparation of this book: to Drs. I. Whimster and J. Burston for much of the material for the Chapters on Skin and Central Nervous System respectively; to Dr. D. Lovell for help with the preparation of the manuscript; and above all to Dr. J. R. Tighe, who not only provided sections of many lesions but also gave a great deal of useful advice at all stages of production of the book. I also wish to express my thanks to the following for lending me sections: Prof. J. Gough, pulmonary alveolar proteinosis; Prof. G. L. Montgomery, primary syphilitic sore; Dr. D. J. O'Brien, cytomegalic inclusion disease; Prof. H. Spencer, Caplan lesion of lung, kaolin pneumoconiosis and Hamman-Rich lung.

Most of the histological sections were prepared by my Chief Technician, A. E. Clark, and by D. Lane. The films were processed by V. Clark, with the assistance of R. Lack. Miss Mary Austin and Miss Jacqueline Stone provided secretarial help. To all these I am greatly indebted.

Great care and skill have been devoted by Schwitter A.G., Basle, to the engraving and by Arts graphiques Coop Suisse, Basle, to the printing of the reproductions. This work has been carried out under the guidance and supervision of Harvey Miller, who has long experience of high-fidelity colour reproduction and whom I wish to thank particularly for his great interest.

R.C.C.

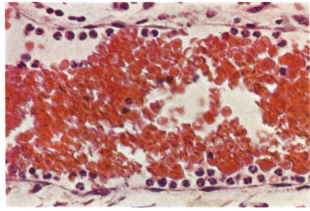

1.1 Acute inflammation: 'pavementing' of endothelium

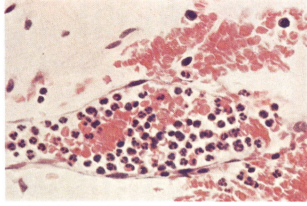

1.2 Acute inflammation: capillary haemorrhage (diapedesis)

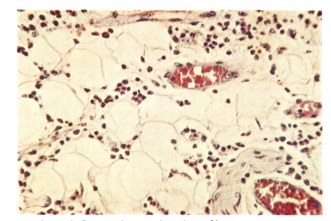

1.3 Acute inflammation: emigration of leucocytes

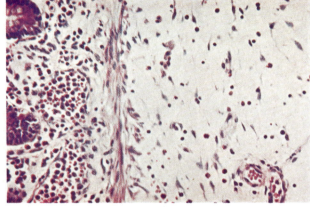

1.4 Inflammatory oedema

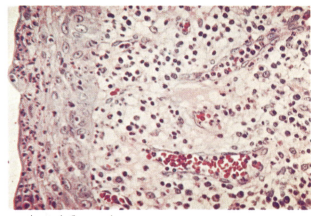

1.5 Acute inflammation

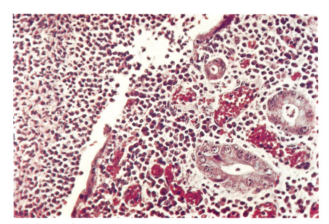

1.6 Acute abscess

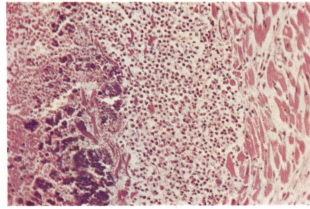

1.7 Pyaemic abscess

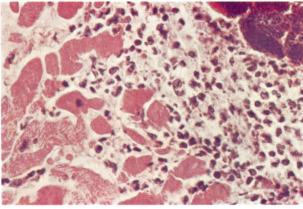

1.8 Pyaemic abscess

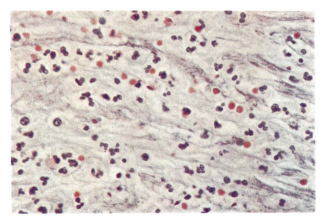

1.9 Acute inflammation: pus

Acute inflammation. 1.1–1.3 illustrate the vascular response that is an essential component of the acute inflammatory reaction. The tissue is the mesentery of an acutely inflamed appendix. **1.1 'Pavementing' of endothelium.** The vessel is a capillary. It is enormously dilated, and polymorphs, mostly neutrophil, adhere to the endothelial surface. Adhesion to the endothelium precedes emigration of the cells into the surrounding tissues and towards the source of the inflammatory stimulus. What causes the leucocytes to stick is unknown. It should be noted that emigration of leucocytes often takes place from the post-capillary venules rather than from the capillaries themselves. This vessel is so dilated that stasis has probably already ensued. **1.2 Capillary haemorrhage (diapedesis of red cells).** The capillary is greatly dilated and the lumen contains numerous polymorphs. The endothelial wall has ruptured and haemorrhage has occurred into the adjacent loose connective tissues. **1.3 Emigration of leucocytes.** Inflammatory cells, nearly all neutrophil polymorphs, have left the dilated vessels and migrated into the adjacent tissues. A nerve fibre is present (bottom right). 1.4–1.6 are from a case of regional enteritis (Crohn's disease). **1.4 Inflammatory oedema.** This section is from the terminal ileum; the crypts of two intestinal glands are visible on the left. The tissues are hyperaemic and some of the dilated capillaries contain many polymorphs. The amount of oedema is striking and is seen most clearly to the right of the muscularis mucosae where the connective tissue cells have been forced apart by the fluid and the inflammatory cells appear to be suspended in clear spaces. **1.5 Acute inflammation.** This shows the acutely inflamed mucosa of the anal canal. There is hyperaemia, and polymorphs are numerous in the dilated capillaries. Polymorphs are also mi-

grating through the stratified squamous epithelium (left) in large numbers. There is considerable inflammatory oedema. The condition had been present for some months and there are some plasma cells and lymphocytes. **1.6 Acute abscess.** An abscess is a collection of pus within the tissues and is produced by an irritant (bacterial or chemical) that is intense but remains localised. Since abscess formation is always accompanied by destruction of tissue, healing results in scar formation. This lesion is in the caecum. There is hyperaemia and an acute abscess (left) has formed deep to the colonic glands (right). The pus filling the abscess consists largely of polymorphs, many of them necrotic and disintegrating. Plasma cells (centre and top right) are numerous around the abscess. **1.7 and 1.8 Pyaemic abscess.** In pyaemia, infection reaches the tissues by the bloodstream from a primary focus elsewhere and multiple abscesses may be formed. **1.7** This lesion is in the myocardium. The abscess contains necrotic cell debris, colonies of staphylococci (left), and large numbers of polymorphs (centre), many of them degenerate. The myocardium is visible on the right. **1.8** A higher power view of another abscess shows that although the myocardial fibres furthest away (bottom left) from the abscess are intact, the fibres nearer the abscess are necrotic, being deeply eosinophilic and lacking nuclei. Most of the polymorphs also are necrotic. Like the myocardial fibres they have been killed by toxins from the staphylococci. **1.9 Acute inflammation: pus.** This is a smear of pus from an acute abscess. It shows strands of fibrin, neutrophil polymorphs, red cells and a few macrophages. No microorganisms are visible in this field, but a Gram stain would probably reveal them.

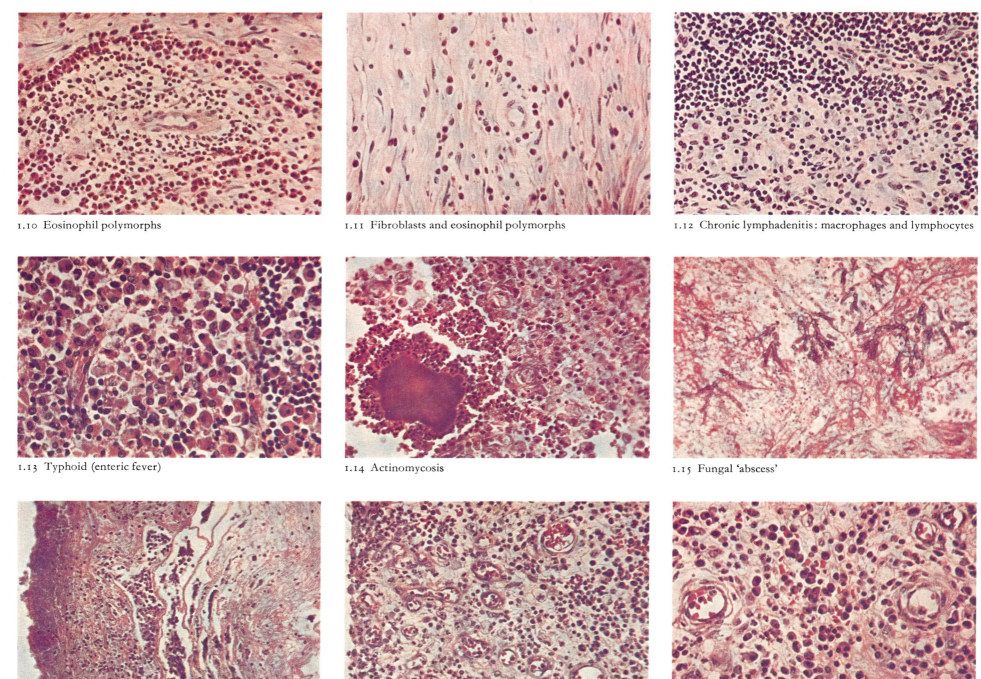

1.10 Eosinophil polymorphs

1.11 Fibroblasts and eosinophil polymorphs

1.12 Chronic lymphadenitis: macrophages and lymphocytes

1.13 Typhoid (enteric fever)

1.14 Actinomycosis

1.15 Fungal 'abscess'

1.16 Pseudomembranous inflammation: diphtheria

1.17 Granulation tissue (repair tissue)

1.18 Granulation tissue

1.10 Eosinophil polymorphs. This shows part of the capsule around an adult filarial worm (*Onchocerca volvulus*). The cells nearest the vessel (centre) are lymphocytes and plasma cells but most of the other cells are eosinophil polymorphs. The presence of many eosinophil polymorphs is often a feature of the tissue response to parasites of this type. **1.11 Fibroblasts and eosinophil polymorphs.** This is another part of the lesion shown in 1.10. Here the capsule consists of collagenous fibrous tissue produced by the many elongated fibroblasts present. There are also numerous eosinophil polymorphs. **1.12 Chronic lymphadenitis: macrophages and lymphocytes.** This is the periphery of a lymph node showing mild reactive changes. The peripheral sinus (bottom half) is distended with phagocytic mononuclear cells, derived from lining cells. The tissue at the top is intersinusoidal and consists of lymphocytes and a few plasma cells. The vessel (top right) is a small venule. **1.13 Typhoid (enteric fever).** In this disease the inflammatory reaction in the tissues is characterised by the presence of large numbers of macrophages and an absence of polymorphs. In this Peyer's patch, macrophages have almost completely displaced the lymphocytes normally present. A few of the macrophages are degenerate but necrosis is not yet pronounced. The cytoplasm of the macrophages is uncharacteristically eosinophilic in this section. **1.14 Actinomycosis.** This is a 'sulphur granule', from an abscess which was located in the appendix region: a colony of *Actinomyces israeli* (left) is surrounded by necrotic debris and polymorphs, and foamy (lipid-laden) macrophages are pres-

ent at the periphery (right). In this form of the disease, infection may spread by the portal vein, to form a 'honeycomb' abscess in the liver. **1.15 Fungal 'abscess'.** This was an incidental finding in the thyroid gland at necropsy of a subject of 16 who had had Hodgkin's disease and had been treated with chemotherapeutic agents which had effectively inhibited the body's defence mechanisms. Branching tubular filaments of *Aspergillus flavus* are growing in dead tissue and fibrin but there is a noteworthy lack of cellular response to them. **1.16 Pseudomembranous inflammation: diphtheria.** In diphtheria, the bacilli remain at the surface and exert their systemic effects by means of exotoxins. This shows a section of a membrane from the tonsil. It consists of bacilli (left, surface), fibrin strands and inflammatory cells (centre), and necrotic epithelium (right). **1.17 and 1.18 Granulation tissue (repair tissue).** Granulation tissue derives its name from the granular appearance of the tissue that fills the gap in the tissues in healing wounds and ulcers. 'Repair tissue' is a less confusing term. **1.17** This shows repair tissue that has enclosed a pelvic abscess. It consists of thick-walled capillary loops and many inflammatory cells, mainly polymorphs and plasma cells. Macrophages are often abundant in granulation tissue. As repair proceeds, fibroblasts appear in increasing numbers and the end-result is a vascular fibrous tissue. **1.18** The thick-walled capillaries, polymorphs, lymphocytes and many plasma cells are seen here in greater detail. The delicate pink-staining fibrils between the inflammatory cells are probably young collagen fibrils.

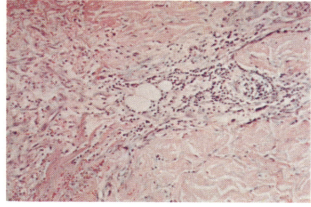

1.19 Healing wound: skin

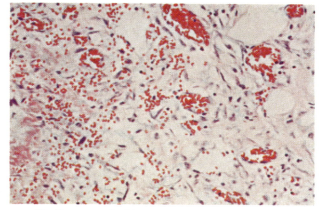

1.20 Healing wound: skin

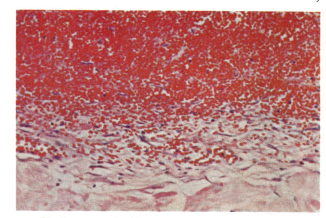

1.21 Healing wound: skin

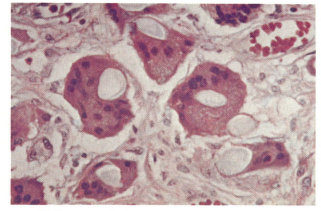

1.22 Healing wound: skin

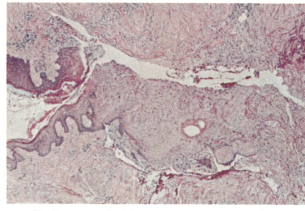

1.23 Healing wound: skin

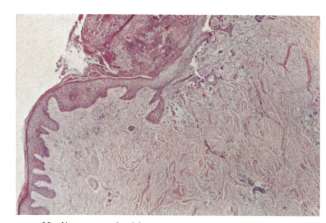

1.24 Healing wound: skin

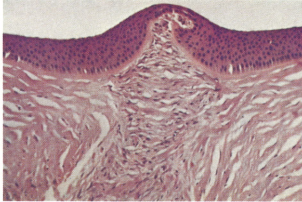

1.25 Healed wound: cornea

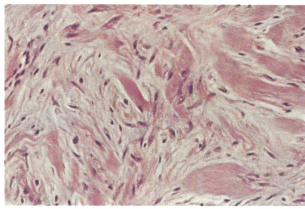

1.26 Keloid

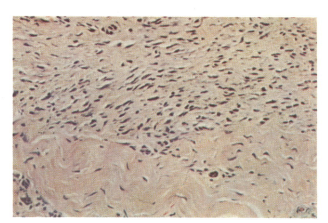

1.27 Fibromatosis

1.19–1.24 Healing wound: skin. 1.19 This is a 10-day surgical wound of skin. Only the dermal part of the wound is visible, the epithelial surface being out of the picture to the left (see 1.23). In the pink-staining dermal collagenous tissues the wound forms a gap which is filled with a paler-staining cellular tissue: closer examination of this would show that it consists of small vessels (mainly dilated capillaries), macrophages, fibroblasts and lymphocytes. **1.20** This is a higher-power view of the same lesion as 1.19 showing some of the widely dilated capillaries and venules. There are also elongated fibroblasts, and macrophages are phagocytosing pink-staining fibrin (left). Extravasated red cells are still present. **1.21** Imperfect haemostasis has led to the formation of a haematoma in this surgical wound. Macrophages are invading the mass of red cells and fibroblasts are active in the collagenous tissues adjacent to it. The fibroblasts are orientated parallel to the mass. **1.22** In this wound, suture material (nylon) implanted during a previous operation has been phagocytosed by multinucleated ('foreign-body') giant cells. Each strand of suture material is surrounded by, or is within, a giant cell. Fibrous tissue is present between the giant cells. **1.23** This is the same wound as in 1.19 and 1.20. The breach in the squamous epithelium is visible on the left, and from the lower edge a mass of new pale-staining squamous epithelial cells has proliferated down into the wound, more or less filling it (centre and right of centre). A gap containing red blood cells separates the mass of epithelial cells on both sides from the dermal connective tissues. Migration of epithelial cells into a wound is an undesirable complication and delays healing. **1.24** This is a 17-day healing surgical wound. The skin epithelium, with its normal interpapillary processes, is visible at the lower left surface. A layer of new squamous epithelium lacking interpapillary processes extends from it to the right and upwards, to cover the healing wound, just visible in the top right quadrant. The new epithelium has migrated underneath a scab (top centre). On close examination the scab would be found to consist of fibrin, inflammatory cells and necrotic epithelium. **1.25 Healed wound: cornea.** The cornea had been incised surgically during an operation two months before the eye was removed. The epithelium covering the healed wound (top centre) is thin and less highly differentiated than the normal epithelium. The gap created in the corneal stroma by the wound is filled with cellular connective tissue (centre) but the breach in Bowman's membrane is still visible under the new epithelium. **1.26 Keloid.** In this healed wound of skin, keloid tissue has formed: this is characterised by the presence of abnormally large collagen fibres (right third) and very large fibroblasts. These cells should be compared with the few very much smaller normal fibroblasts present, and with the cells in 1.27. **1.27 Fibromatosis.** This is from a lesion of the palmar fascia. The collagen-forming fibroblasts (top half) have much larger nuclei than the inactive 'fibrocytes' in the normal mature collagen (bottom half). The cells exhibit equally striking differences in cytoplasmic content and structure but these are not visible here. In fibromatosis the fibroblasts may be so numerous and 'active-looking' as to suggest neoplasia but the lesion is benign and eventually becomes quiescent.

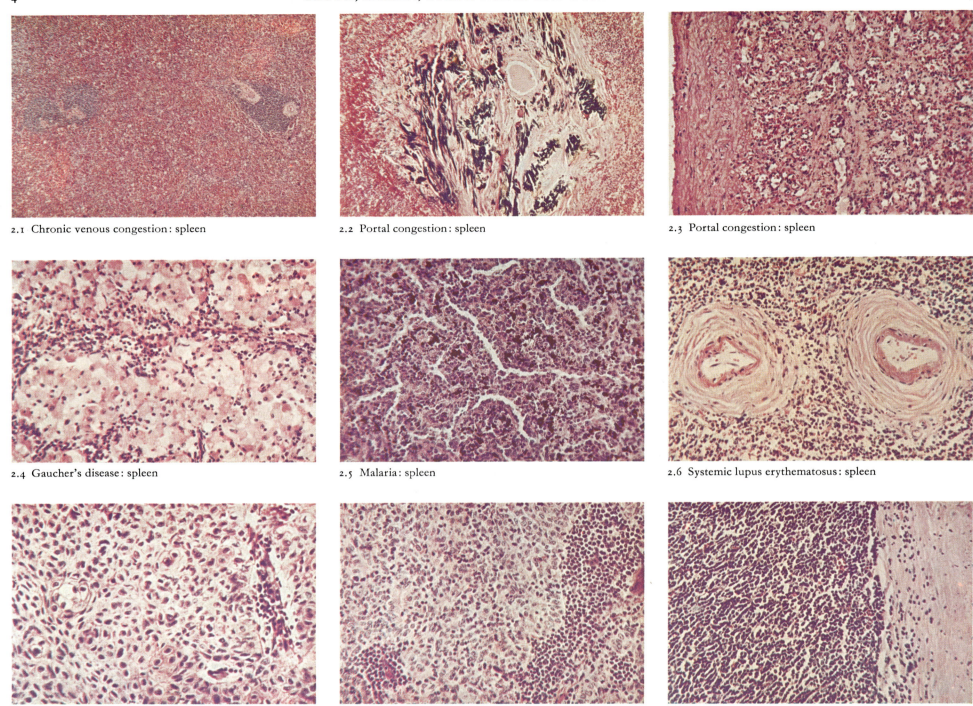

2.1 Chronic venous congestion: spleen

2.2 Portal congestion: spleen

2.3 Portal congestion: spleen

2.4 Gaucher's disease: spleen

2.5 Malaria: spleen

2.6 Systemic lupus erythematosus: spleen

2.7 Thymoma

2.8 Thymoma

2.9 Thymoma

2.1 Chronic venous congestion: spleen. Macroscopically this was a dark red, rubbery 'cricket-ball' spleen. The splenic sinuses are full of blood and the Malpighian corpuscles are small and atrophic. **2.2** and **2.3 Portal congestion: spleen.** The spleen was moderately enlarged and the thickened capsule was adherent to the neighbouring tissues. The cut surface was 'meaty' in appearance. **2.2** This is a 'tobacco nodule' or Gamma-Gandy body which was visible as a brown spot on the cut surface. It consists of dense fibrous tissue impregnated with deeply basophilic iron salts. Siderotic nodules are the result of organisation or break-down of blood repeatedly extravasated from the congested splenic vessels and haemorrhage is still visible (left) round the lesion. **2.3** The sinuses are prominent, the pulp is fibrosed, and the capsule (left) is slightly thickened. A small haemorrhage is present (right). **2.4 Gaucher's disease: spleen.** The organ is packed with large cells whose cytoplasm is full of lipid (kerasin) and consequently appears foamy. The cells, part of the reticuloendothelial system, are found both inside and outside the sinusoids. There is atrophy of the splenic lymphoid tissue including the Malpighian corpuscles. **2.5 Malaria: spleen.** The sinusoids and their lining cells are prominent. In the intersinusoidal tissue, which shows fibrosis, there are many pigment-laden phagocytes. Sometimes the pigment is present in the endothelium. It is haematin, produced from haemoglobin by the malaria para-

site and increased in long-standing cases. **2.6 Systemic lupus erythematosus: spleen.** Vascular lesions are prominent in this disease in which there may be widespread and progressive degeneration of the connective tissues. Here there is great increase in fibrous tissue around two penicillary arteries. The collagen is arranged in concentric lamellae: 'onion-skinning'. There is also deposition of eosinophilic material in the intima. Sometimes the vessels show fibrinoid necrosis. **2.7–2.9 Thymoma.** Thymomas are probably the commonest tumours of the anterior mediastinum. They are usually benign, often lobulated, and enclosed in a fibrous capsule. Thymomas are composed of varying proportions of epithelial cells and thymocytes (lymphocytes). In some tumours one cell type predominates to the almost complete exclusion of the other. **2.7** This tumour consists of large, pale epithelial cells which have large nuclei and prominent nucleoli. The cells' boundaries are ill-defined. Some cells are forming a rudimentary Hassall corpuscle (left). The stroma (right) is infiltrated with lymphocytes. **2.8** This lesion also is epithelial but lymphocytes are present not only in the stroma but also mingled with the epithelial cells. Tumours of this type may resemble a dysgerminoma or seminoma. Thymomas of epithelial cell type are sometimes associated with myasthenia gravis. **2.9** This tumour consists of small mature lymphocytes and it is enclosed within a thick fibrous capsule (right).

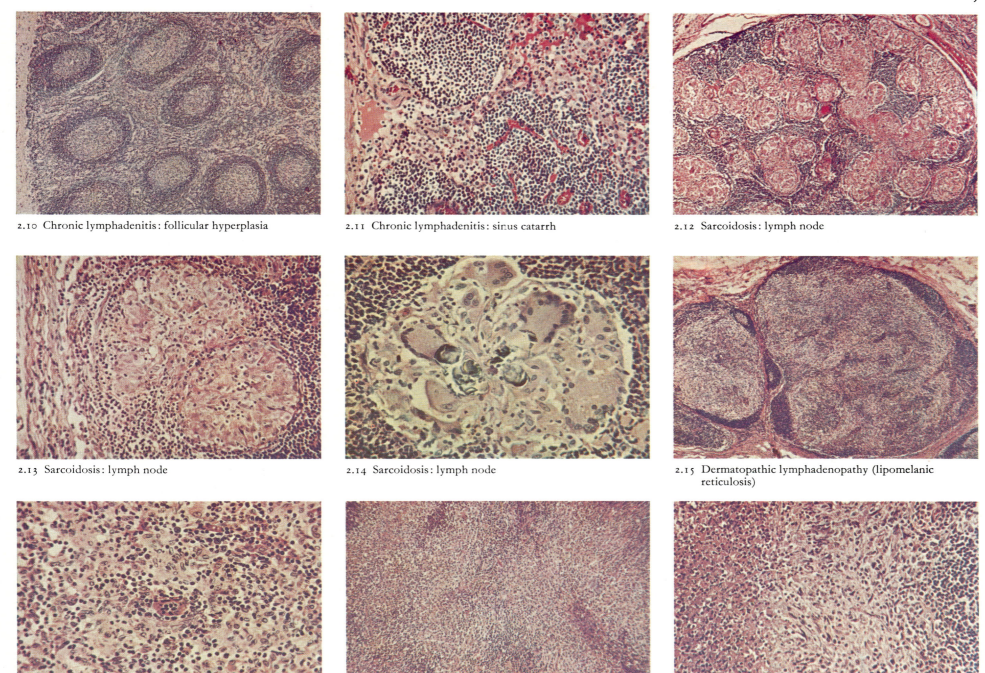

2.10 Chronic lymphadenitis: follicular hyperplasia

2.11 Chronic lymphadenitis: sinus catarrh

2.12 Sarcoidosis: lymph node

2.13 Sarcoidosis: lymph node

2.14 Sarcoidosis: lymph node

2.15 Dermatopathic lymphadenopathy (lipomelanic reticulosis)

2.16 Dermatopathic lymphadenopathy (lipomelanic reticulosis)

2.17 Cat scratch disease: lymph node

2.18 Cat scratch disease: lymph node

2.10 and 2.11 Chronic lymphadenitis. 2.10 Follicular hyperplasia. There is increase in numbers of follicles and enlargement of the germinal centres in the cortex of the node. High power examination shows many mitotic figures inside germinal centres and phagocytes ingesting cell debris are also often present. The presence of follicles in the medulla is frequent in follicular lymphomas but it is not diagnostic of this lesion. **2.11 Sinus catarrh.** In this node the reaction mainly affects the sinuses which are distended with lymph and a large number of mononuclear cells (macrophages) derived from the lining cells. The intersinusoidal tissue is hyperaemic. The capsule and subcapsular sinus are on the left. **2.12–2.14 Sarcoidosis: lymph node.** Sarcoidosis is a clinical syndrome of unknown aetiology. The granulomatous sarcoid reaction is non-specific and can be elicited by a variety of agents, for example beryllium. It is also occasionally seen in lymph nodes draining a carcinoma. **2.12** This lymph node from a patient with sarcoidosis has been largely replaced by granulomata. **2.13** Two small granulomata composed almost entirely of altered histiocytes (epithelioid cells) are located close to the capsule of the node (left). There is no necrosis. Identical follicles are found in proliferative non-caseating tuberculosis and in fact tubercle follicles usually start beneath the capsule because the tubercle bacilli usually enter the node via the subcapsular sinus. **2.14** In this granuloma most of the cells are

giant and multinucleated and some (centre) contain laminated basophilic inclusion bodies (Schaumann bodies). These are very dense and calcified and have fragmented on sectioning. One small asteroid is present (top centre). When the lesions in sarcoidosis involute the histiocytes appear to change into fibroblasts and the end-result is fibrous replacement. **2.15** and **2.16 Dermatopathic lymphadenopathy (lipomelanic reticulosis).** This affects lymph nodes draining chronically inflamed skin (e.g. eczema or psoriasis). The nodes are enlarged but the architecture is preserved. **2.15** There is great hyperplasia of the intersinusoidal tissue which is sufficient to compress the follicles at the periphery of the node. **2.16** It is easy to mistake this lesion for a lymphoma but the hyperplastic reticulum cells are very uniform and abnormal cells are lacking. Lymphocytes are scattered among them. Often the reticulum cells contain melanin, haemosiderin and finely divided fat. **2.17** and **2.18 Cat scratch disease: lymph node.** This is caused by a virus. **2.17** The node contains irregular sinuous abscesses filled with necrotic debris and surrounded by elongated palisaded histiocytes (epithelioid cells). **2.18** The centre of the abscess is on the left. Surrounding it is a zone of histiocytes (centre) which are elongated and show a tendency to palisading and outside these (right) are the lymphocytes of the node. The histological appearances in cat scratch disease are the same as in lymphogranuloma venereum.

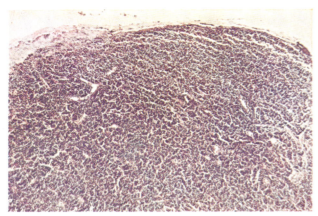

2.19   Malignant lymphoma, lymphocytic type, well-differentiated (lymphosarcoma): lymph node

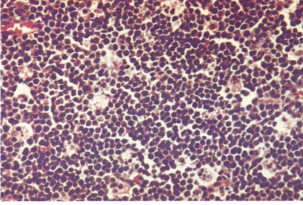

2.20   Malignant lymphoma, lymphocytic type, well-differentiated (lymphosarcoma): lymph node

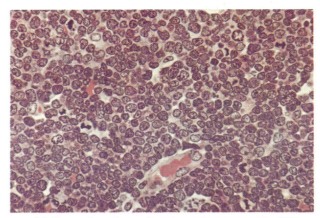

2.21   Malignant lymphoma, lymphocytic type, poorly differentiated (lymphosarcoma, lymphoblastoma): lymph node

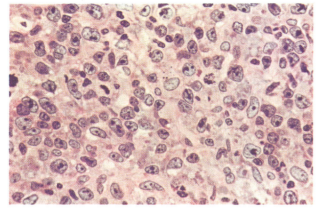

2.22   Malignant lymphoma, histiocytic type (reticulum cell sarcoma): skin

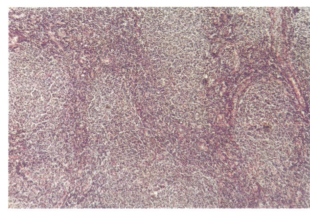

2.23   Malignant lymphoma, lymphocytic type, nodular (follicular lymphoma, Brill-Symmers' disease): lymph node

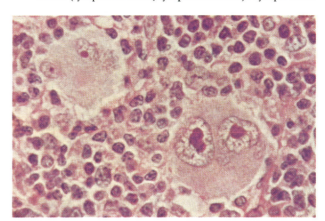

2.24   Hodgkin's disease, lymphocytic predominance (Hodgkin's paragranuloma): lymph node

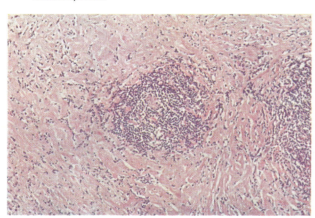

2.25   Hodgkin's disease, nodular sclerosing type: lymph node.

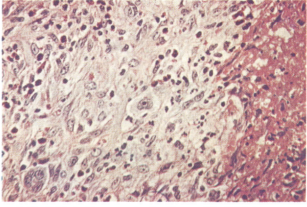

2.26   Hodgkin's disease, mixed cell type (Hodgkin's granuloma): lymph node.

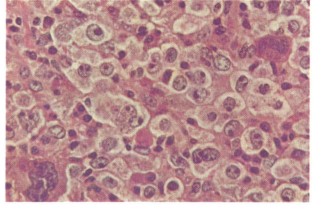

2.27   Hodgkin's disease, reticular type (Hodgkin's sarcoma): lymph node

2.19–2.27 Malignant lymphoma. 2.19 –, lymphocytic type, well-differentiated (lympho-sarcoma): lymph node. The node is replaced by a uniform mass of small lymphocytes, obliterating all normal lymph node architecture. **2.20 –, lymphocytic type, well-differentiated (lymphosarcoma): lymph node.** This is a higher-power view of lesion similar to 2.19, showing the neoplastic small lymphocytes in more detail. It also shows the presence of occasional phagocytic histiocytes between the tumour cells. **2.21 –, lymphocytic type, poorly differentiated (lymphosarcoma, lymphoblastoma): lymph node.** The tumour is composed of sheets of immature lymphoid cells. These differ from the cells in 2.20 in showing more frequent mitoses and in having a more open 'vesicular' nucleus. This illustration has been taken from a thin (0.5 μm) section to demonstrate the detailed structure of the cells more clearly. **2.22 –, histiocytic type (reticulum cell sarcoma): skin.** This also is from a thin (0.5 μm) section. The lesion, a cutaneous deposit, is composed of rather pleomorphic cells with open, vesicular nuclei, and ill-defined cytoplasmic borders. Many of the nuclei are elongated or reniform. **2.23 –, lymphocytic type, nodular (follicular lymphoma, Brill-Symmers' disease): lymph node.** The tumour is composed of lymphoid cells that are forming a nodular or follicular pattern. These follicles are much less well-defined than those in reactive follicular hyperplasia. **2.24 Hodgkin's**

disease, lymphocytic predominance (Hodgkin's paragranuloma): lymph node. A typical Reed-Sternberg cell with a 'mirror-image' double nucleus is present (bottom right). Each of the nuclei contains a very prominent eosinophilic nucleolus. Apart from the other large cell (top left), the remaining cells are predominantly small lymphocytes. **2.25 Hodgkin's disease, nodular sclerosing type: lymph node.** The central island of cellular Hodgkin's tissue is surrounded by dense collagen, the edge of another cellular focus being visible on the right. In this type of lymphoma, the bulk of the node often consists of collagenous tissue. **2.26 Hodgkin's disease, mixed cell type (Hodgkin's granuloma): lymph node.** The tumour is composed of histiocytes, polymorphs (including many eosinophils e.g. at top left), and Reed-Sternberg cells (e.g. at lower left corner). A few small lymphocytes are present. The deeply eosinophilic tissue on the right is necrotic. **2.27 Hodgkin's disease, reticular type (Hodgkin's sarcoma): lymph node.** The node is replaced by large pleomorphic cells some of which are multinucleate and resemble Reed-Sternberg cells (e.g. left of centre and lower left corner). There are few lymphocytes or inflammatory cells. In general, in Hodgkin's disease the lymphocyte-predominance and nodular-sclerosing types are associated with a better prognosis than the mixed-cellularity and reticular types (lymphocyte depletion).

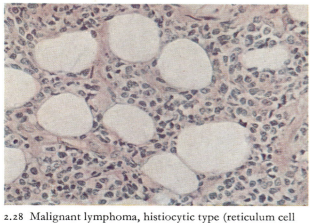

2.28 Malignant lymphoma, histiocytic type (reticulum cell sarcoma)

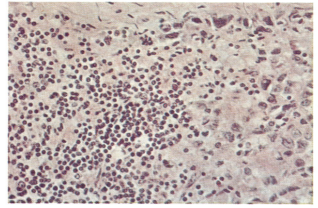

2.29 Secondary carcinoma: lymph node

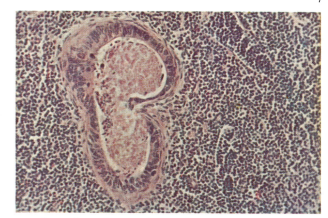

2.30 Secondary adenocarcinoma: lymph node

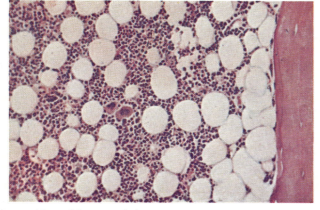

2.31 Normal haemopoietic marrow

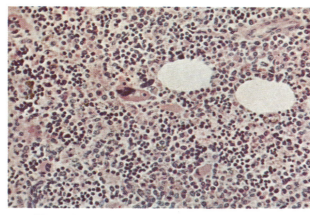

2.32 Hyperplasia of haemopoietic marrow

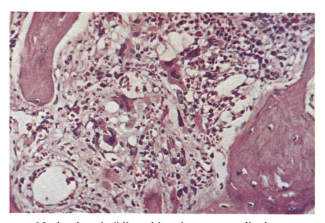

2.33 Myelosclerosis (idiopathic primary generalised myelofibrosis): marrow

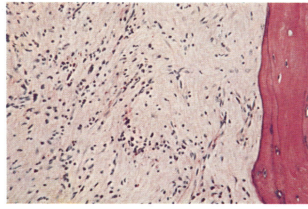

2.34 Myelosclerosis: marrow

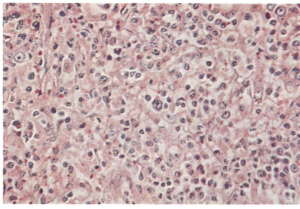

2.35 Myelosclerosis: spleen

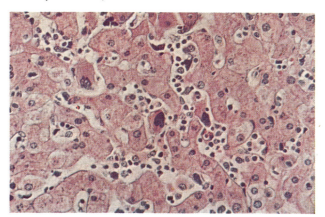

2.36 Extramedullary haemopoiesis: liver

2.28 Malignant lymphoma, histiocytic type (reticulum cell sarcoma). This shows reticulum cells invading the fatty tissues around a lymph node. **2.29 Secondary carcinoma: lymph node.** Tumour cells (right) are growing into the node from the subcapsular sinus (top). The malignant nature of the cells which are undifferentiated is evident in the pronounced basophilia and pleomorphism of the nuclei. The peripheral sinus is the point of arrival of lymph and therefore of carcinomatous emboli. Small deposits of tumours are easily overlooked or mistaken for sinus hyperplasia. Secondary deposits usually have the same features as the primary. **2.30 Secondary adenocarcinoma: lymph node.** This secondary deposit is deep within the node. It consists of a large acinus, lined by very abnormal columnar epithelial cells and filled with necrotic material. Round it is a small amount of fibrous stroma. Two sinuses are packed with lymphocytes. The primary tumour was in the stomach. **2.31 Normal haemopoietic marrow.** This shows the relative proportions between fat and haemopoietic tissue that normally exists in the marrow in the vertebral bodies. Among the haemopoietic cells are white cell precursors, red cell precursors and megakaryocytes. Flattened inactive osteoblasts cover the lamellar bone on the right. **2.32 Hyperplasia of haemopoietic marrow.** There is less fat and more haemopoietic tissue. The haemopoietic elements are normal. The more numerous darker-staining clusters are red cell precursors and the less densely-staining groups are leukocyte precursors including many myeloblasts. There are also

megakaryocytes and haemosiderin-containing macrophages. **2.33–2.35 Myelosclerosis (idiopathic primary generalised myelofibrosis).** This is probably related to myeloid leukaemia and polycythaemia vera, all three being 'myeloproliferative disorders'. In **2.33** the bone marrow has been replaced by loose connective tissue in which megakaryocytes and abnormal reticulum cells are prominent. The increase of megakaryocytes is a characteristic feature of myelosclerosis. **2.34** shows a more advanced degree of fibrosis of the bone marrow. The haemopoietic cells have been completely replaced by delicate connective tissue in which there are fibroblasts, plasma cells and lymphocytes. **2.35** This is a section of the spleen. The organ was dark brownish red in colour and weighed 820 g. It consists of intensely cellular tissue in which abnormal reticulum cells are prominent. There are also many immature cells, probably erythrocyte and leukocyte precursors. An increase of reticulin could be demonstrated but in the marrow this increase was proportionately much greater (2.34). The Malpighian bodies were atrophic. **2.36 Extramedullary haemopoiesis: liver.** This is the liver of an infant which died of haemolytic disease of the newborn (erythroblastosis fetalis). The sinusoids contain megakaryocytes and immature red and white cells. The small dark cells are red cell precursors. The liver cells are well-preserved and the glycogen-laden cytoplasm is pale and granular. Extramedullary haemopoiesis is also a feature of myelosclerosis, probably part of the myeloproliferation.

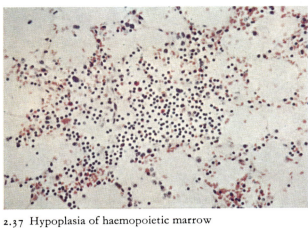

2.37 Hypoplasia of haemopoietic marrow

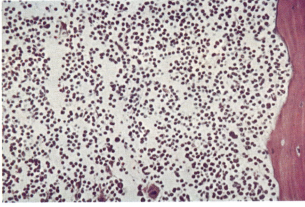

2.38 Malignant lymphoma, lymphocytic type: marrow

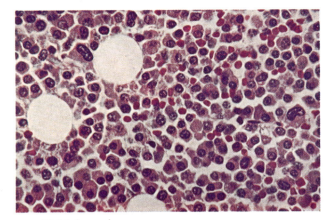

2.39 Multiple myeloma: marrow

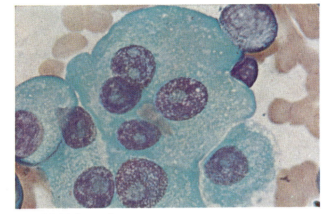

2.40 Multiple myeloma: marrow

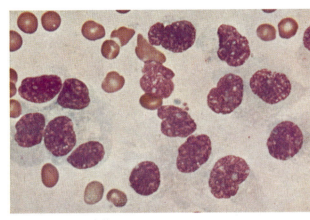

2.41 Carcinoma cells: marrow

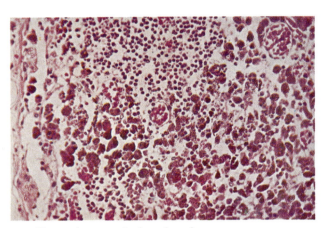

2.42 Haemochromatosis: lymph node

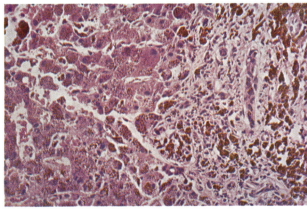

2.43 Haemochromatosis: liver

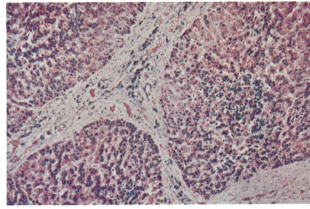

2.44 Haemochromatosis: liver

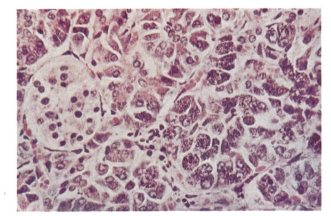

2.45 Haemochromatosis: pancreas

2.37 Hypoplasia of haemopoietic marrow. This is the vertebral marrow from a case of Hodgkin's disease treated with nitrogen mustard and in whom aplastic anaemia developed. The haemopoietic tissue has been destroyed and apart from the fat there remains only a scanty population of plasma cells, lymphocytes, eosinophils and megakaryocytes. Some haemorrhage has occurred.
2.38 Malignant lymphoma, lymphocytic type: marrow. Apart from a megakaryocyte (bottom centre) the haemopoietic tissue has been replaced by small mature lymphocytes. The bone trabecula (right) is being eroded, apparently by the tumour cells. This degree of involvement of the marrow usually denotes lymphocytic leukaemia rather than lymphosarcoma. **2.39** and **2.40 Multiple myeloma: marrow.** This is a highly malignant primary tumour of bone marrow. It is located in red marrow sites (vertebrae, skull, ribs and ends of long bones) and consists of multiple soft red nodules which cause destruction of the bone and therefore a characteristic x-ray picture. Sometimes it is diffuse. **2.39** In this section the marrow is replaced by plasma cells some of which appear abnormal. Characteristically the nucleus is at one pole of the cell. Some of the nuclei also show the 'clock-face' chromatin pattern clearly, and the abundant cytoplasm is typically amphophilic. This bluish-pink colour is produced by the abundant ribosomal ribonucleoprotein in the cytoplasm taking up some haematoxylin. The ribosomes are concerned with formation of the globulins found in the serum. Mitoses are rarely seen. **2.40** This is a smear stained with Leishman's stain. The cells are primitive plasma cells, one having multiple nuclei. The nucleoli are large and sometimes multiple, the cytoplasm is basophilic, and a perinuclear 'halo' is evident (on left, for example). The high nucleolus/nucleus ratio helps to distinguish myeloma from benign plasmacytic reactions. The erythrocytes form rouleaux due to alteration in the serum proteins. **2.41 Carcinoma cells: marrow.** This is a marrow smear, stained with Leishman's stain, from a

patient who had had an undifferentiated carcinoma of breast. It shows scattered groups of cells which possess very primitive nuclei with delicate chromatin strands and several prominent nucleoli. The abundant very pale-staining cytoplasm is ill-defined and some of the cells form syncytial aggregates. **2.42–2.45 Haemochromatosis.** In haemochromatosis excess iron is absorbed and stored as haemosiderin, mostly in the parenchymatous and epithelial cells, the amount of iron stored being many times normal. There is relatively little in the reticulo-endothelial system, in contrast with transfusional siderosis. **2.42** This is a lymph node. The sinuses are full of haemosiderin-laden macrophages but there is no fibrosis. The capsule and subcapsular sinus are on the left. **2.43** The liver shows portal cirrhosis and fibrosis tissue is greatly increased around the bile-duct (right). There are many haemosiderin-laden macrophages in the fibrous tissue and the same pigment is present in high concentration in the parenchymal cells (centre and left). Pigment deposition precedes the cirrhotic process. In contrast, even in advanced siderosis, for example after multiple transfusions, the large amounts of haemosiderin that accumulate in the liver rarely cause fibrosis and cirrhosis. **2.44** This section of the cirrhotic liver has been stained by the Prussian blue method to demonstrate the iron of the haemosiderin. The pigment is abundant within the liver cells as well as in macrophages in the broad bands of dense fibrous tissue which divide the parenchymal cells into regeneration nodules of various sizes. **2.45** In the pancreas most of the haemosiderin is within the cells of the exocrine tissue though refractile granules are visible in the cytoplasm of the islet cells (left). In advanced lesions both exocrine and endocrine tissues may be destroyed and loss of the beta cells produces diabetes mellitus. Haemosiderin, melanin, and haemofuscin (a non-iron containing pigment) are deposited in the skin and so the condition is sometimes termed 'bronze diabetes'.

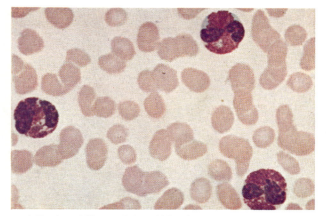

2.46 Eosinophilia: peripheral blood

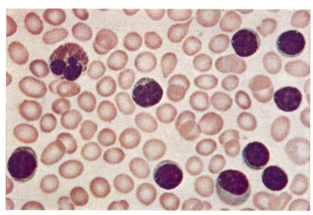

2.47 Chronic lymphocytic leukaemia: peripheral blood

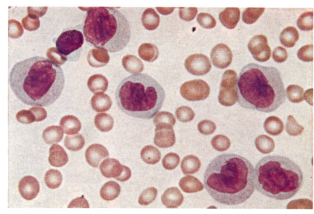

2.48 Monocytic leukaemia (Schilling type): peripheral blood

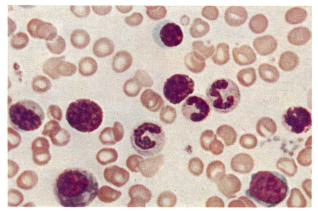

2.49 Chronic granulocytic leukaemia: peripheral blood

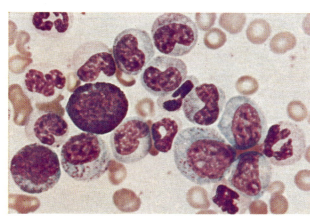

2.50 Chronic granulocytic leukaemia: marrow

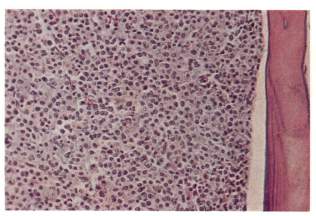

2.51 Acute granulocytic leukaemia: marrow

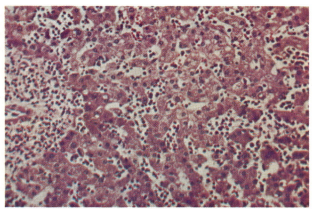

2.52 Chronic granulocytic leukaemia: liver

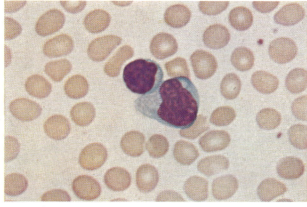

2.53 Infectious mononucleosis (glandular fever):
peripheral blood

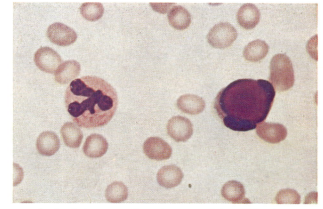

2.54 Systemic lupus erythematosus: peripheral blood
preparation

In the next two pages the smears of bone marrow and peripheral blood are, with the exception of 2.56 and 2.63, at the same magnification (×1,050), to allow the cells to be compared. All smears have been stained with Leishman's stain. **2.46 Eosinophilia: peripheral blood.** There was considerable increase in the numbers of leucocytes in the peripheral blood and 90% were eosinophils. Three eosinophils are seen in this smear. They are mature and the nucleus is bi-lobed. Eosinophilia is common in allergic disorders, skin diseases, and in parasitic infestation, especially hookworm disease and trichinosis. **2.47 Chronic lymphocytic leukaemia: peripheral blood.** There is a considerable increase in the number of small lymphocytes. One of them is a large lymphocyte. An eosinophil leucocyte is also present (top left). **2.48 Monocytic leukaemia (Schilling type): peripheral blood.** This shows the monocytes present in large numbers in this disease. Each cell has a large 'folded' nucleus and abundant very finely granular cytoplasm. This type of leukaemia is nearly always acute and has many of the clinical features of acute granulocytic leukaemia. **2.49 and 2.50 Chronic granulocytic leukaemia. 2.49** In this smear of the peripheral blood the white cells are greatly increased in number and unsegmented neutrophils predominate. The other cells include an eosinophil (left of centre) and a basophil leucocyte; myelocytes and a myeloblast (bottom right). The leucocytes can be shown to differ from normal leucocytes by the reduction of cytoplasmic alkaline phosphatase. **2.50** In this marrow smear white cell precursors predominate. They include four promyelocytes, with nucleoli; two

myelocytes, one full of basophil granules; seven metamyelocytes; and six neutrophil polymorphs. **2.51 Acute granulocytic leukaemia: marrow.** In this section there is complete replacement of the marrow by large cells of primitive type which are almost all myeloblasts. Darker-staining more mature forms, including polymorphs, are present in small numbers but there are no megakaryocytes. **2.52 Chronic granulocytic leukaemia: liver.** In this section leukaemic cells diffusely infiltrate the organ but tend to congregate in the portal tract (left). The concentration of cells in the portal tract is much less than in chronic lymphocytic leukaemia. **2.53 Infectious mononucleosis (glandular fever): peripheral blood.** The lymphocyte on the right is abnormal. The chromatin of its nucleus is arranged in long strands like skeins of wool whereas in the lymphocyte on the left it forms coarse clumps. The abnormal lymphocyte also has more cytoplasm which is not uniform in texture; it is more 'fluffy' than normal. **2.54 Systemic lupus erythematosus: peripheral blood preparation.** The lupus erythematosus (L.E.) cell (right) is a neutrophil polymorph which contains a very large cytoplasmic inclusion, thought to be chromatin derived from nuclear fragments. The nucleus of the polymorph has been pushed to the periphery. An important feature is the complete loss of chromatin detail which distinguishes the L.E. cell from a tart cell in which chromatin detail persists. The other cell is a neutrophil polymorph.

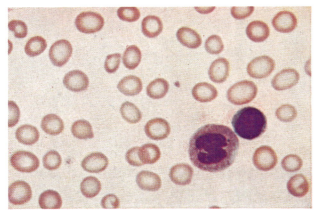

2.55 Iron-deficiency anaemia: peripheral blood

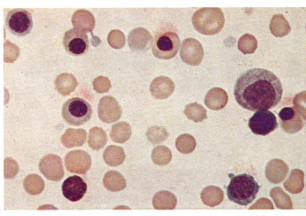

2.56 Haemolytic disease of the new-born (erythroblastosis fetalis): peripheral blood

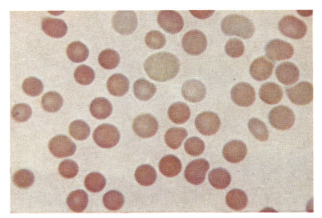

2.57 Congenital spherocytic anaemia: peripheral blood

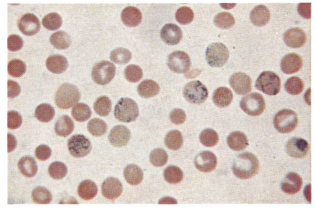

2.58 Congenital spherocytic anaemia: reticulocytes in peripheral blood

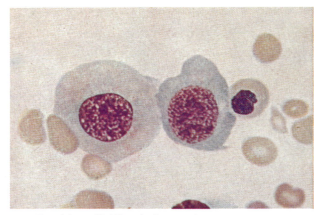

2.59 Pernicious (Addisonian) anaemia: marrow

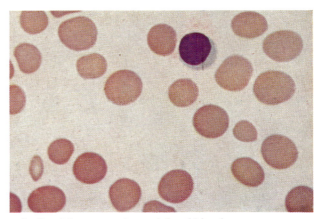

2.60 Pernicious anaemia: peripheral blood

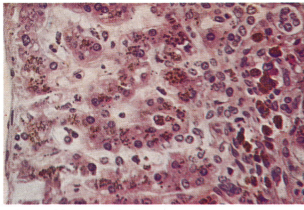

2.61 Pernicious anaemia: liver

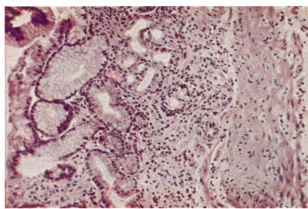

2.62 Pernicious anaemia: stomach

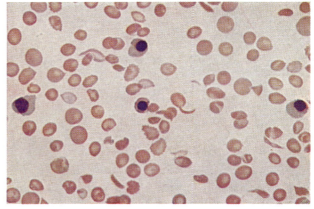

2.63 Sickle cell anaemia: peripheral blood

2.55 Iron-deficiency anaemia: peripheral blood. The erythrocytes are small (microcytic) and they stain poorly (hypochromic), the unstained centre producing a 'ring' appearance. A neutrophil leucocyte, a small lymphocyte, and several platelets are present. **2.56 Haemolytic disease of the new-born (erythroblastosis fetalis): peripheral blood.** The cell in the bottom left corner is a lymphocyte. The largest cell is a myelocyte and beneath it is a basophil normoblast, as is the cell in the bottom right corner. The other five cells are normoblasts: three are polychromatic (top left quadrant) and two are normochromic. The red cells show anisocytosis (variations in size) and macrocytes are present. Some cells show polychromasia. The large number of early red cells is due to the severe haemolysis that affects the baby and which is caused by Rhesus factor incompatibility between mother and baby. **2.57 and 2.58 Congenital spherocytic anaemia. 2.57** In the peripheral blood the red cells are deeply-stained and their average diameter is smaller than normal (microcytes). The few larger cells are slightly polychromatic. **2.58** This smear of peripheral blood has been 'vitally' stained by cresyl violet and then by Leishman's stain. Six of the red cells are reticulocytes. They contain a delicate blue network which is a remnant of the endoplasmic reticulum. Note that the average diameter of these young cells is greater than that of the more mature cells. **2.59–2.62 Pernicious (Addisonian) anaemia: 2.59** This is a marrow smear. The central cell is a basophilic megaloblast. The cell on its left is a polychromatic megaloblast and the third cell is a polychromatic normoblast. The chromatin pattern of the megaloblasts' nuclei is finely reticular compared with **the much** coarser clumps of the normoblast chromatin. The erythrocytes show fairly pronounced **variations** in size (anisocytosis) but their average size is large and they are well filled with haemoglobin. **2.60** In the peripheral blood, the red cells are large (macrocytic) and well-filled with haemoglobin. One has an oval shape (bottom right). Ovalocytosis is often a prominent feature. Anisocytosis is slight in this field. A small lymphocyte is present. **2.61** This section of liver shows a marked increase in the amount of haemosiderin. It is present within phagocytes in the portal tract (right) and also in the liver cells. A little is present within the Kupffer cells. **2.62** This is a section of stomach and it shows atrophy of the gastric mucosa. Oxyntic and parietal cells have disappeared and the surviving cells are mucus-secreting. Plasma cells and lymphocytes infiltrate the mucosa. The muscularis mucosae (right) is much thicker than normal. **2.63 Sickle cell anaemia: peripheral blood.** A significant number of erythrocytes are narrow, elongated and 'sickle-shaped', and 'target' cells are visible. The red cells also show considerable anisocytosis and poikilocytosis. The four nucleated cells are normoblasts and in three of them the cytoplasm is polychromatic. A high proportion of the erythrocytes also exhibit polychromasia. Sickling is not always evident in stained smears, but it affects nearly all of the red cells in sealed wet films when the oxygen tension is reduced. It can also be demonstrated in patients with the sickle cell trait who are characteristically asymptomatic.

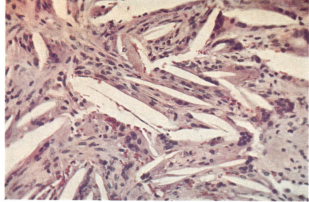
3.1 Cholesteatoma

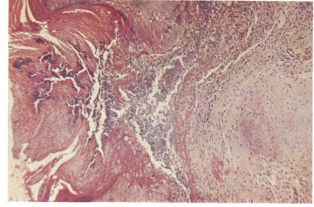
3.2 Chondrodermatitis helicis chronica (perichondritis)

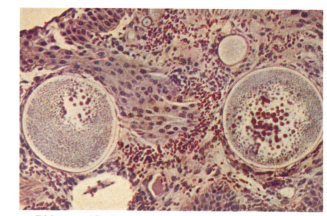
3.3 Rhinosporidiosis

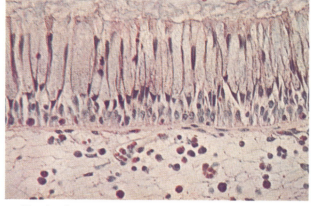
3.4 Nasal polyp

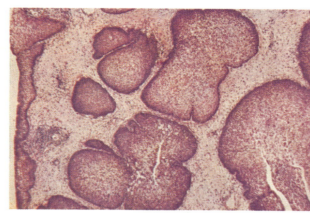
3.5 Nasal polyp: 'inverted papilloma'

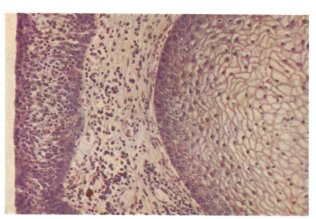
3.6 Nasal polyp: 'inverted papilloma'

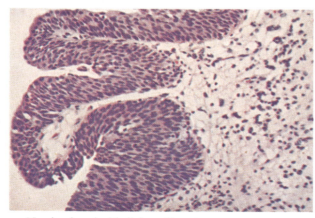
3.7 Nasal polyp: 'epithelial papilloma'

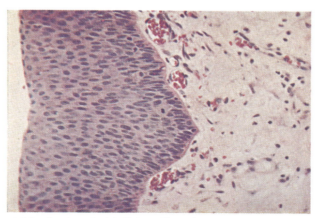
3.8 Nasal polyp: 'epithelial papilloma'

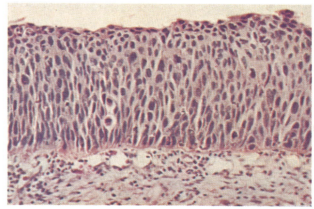
3.9 Nasal polyp: 'epithelial papilloma'

3.1 Cholesteatoma. This serious lesion is usually a sequel of chronic otitis media and mastoid-itis. It is not a true neoplasm but an overgrowth of squamous epithelium within the middle ear. This shows the soft material from the centre of the lesion. It consists of crystals of cholesterol, macrophages and foreign body giant cells. The cholesterol crystals have dissolved during processing of the tissues and only the clefts they occupied remain. Most of the crystals appear to lie within the giant cells. They are derived from old haemorrhage and degenerating squamous epithelial cells growing within the confined space of the inner ear. **3.2 Chondrodermatitis nodularis helicis chronica (perichondritis).** The lesion was a small painful nodule on the border of the helix of the ear. In the centre (left) is a small scab consisting of inspissated keratin. Considerable destruction of the fibro-elastic cartilage (right) of the external ear has occurred and small cysts (centre) are forming beneath the perichondrium. **3.3 Rhinosporidiosis.** This is a fungal infection of the nasal mucous membrane. This is a section of a friable polypoid mass from the nose. Beneath the squamous epithelium lie several spherules full of spores of varying size, the central ones (sporangia) being much larger and deeply eosinophilic. The haemorrhage presumably occurred at operation. **3.4 Nasal polyp.** This was a large, soft, gelatinous mass. The epithelium, covered with mucin, consists of very large mucin-secreting goblet cells and small basal cells. The basement membrane is thick and the very oedematous core is infiltrated by eosin-

ophils, plasma cells and lymphocytes. This lesion is entirely benign. It is not neoplastic but the result of inflammatory oedema. **3.5 and 3.6 Nasal polyp: 'inverted papilloma'. 3.5** This polyp consists of well-differentiated transitional epithelium which forms irregular clefts and spaces. The stroma is loose, oedematous connective tissue which is lightly infiltrated with chronic inflammatory cells. The lesion is often bulky but it is not malignant. **3.6** This is a higher power view of a similar lesion. Though there is considerable inflammation, the surface epithelium being heavily infiltrated by polymorphs and the underlying tissues by plasma cells and lymphocytes, the transitional epithelium is well-differentiated. **3.7–3.9 Nasal polyp: 'epithelial papilloma'.** This form of polyp is more definitely neoplastic, in that it is apt to recur and undergo malignant change. In **3.7** the epithelium is transitional in form but atypical and growing actively, the small dark cells being mitotic figures. Lymphocytes and plasma cells are present in the oedematous core. **3.8** and **3.9** are higher power views of tumours even more active than 3.7. In both the transitional epithelium is very thick and the cells have large basophilic nuclei with prominent nucleoli. The number of mitotic figures is very striking. The cells in 3.9 have lost their normal polarity and are arranged in irregular fashion. Only a few lymphocytes are present in the vascular, oedematous core.

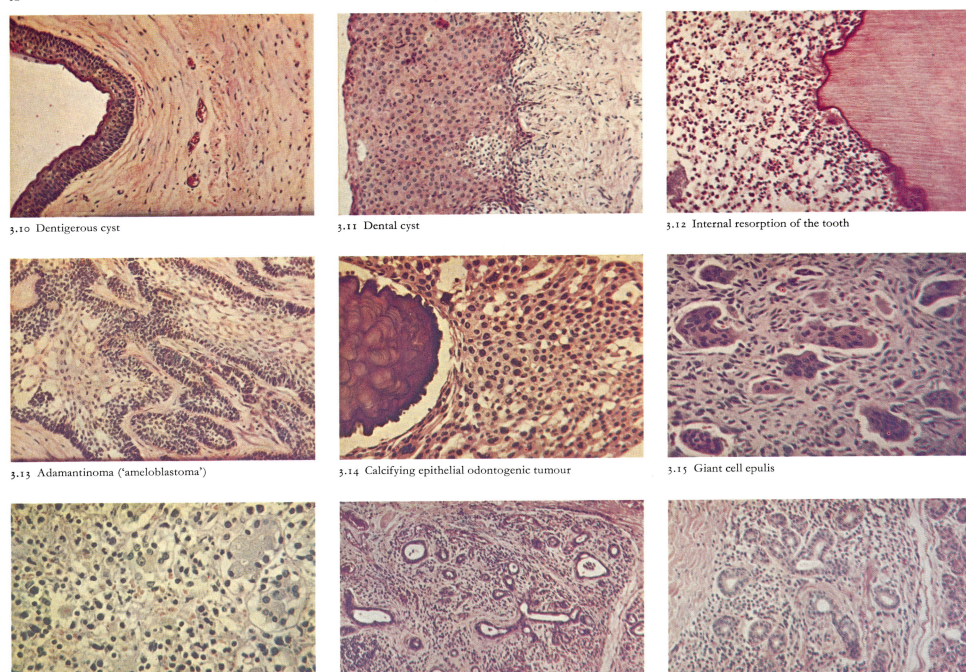

3.10 Dentigerous cyst   3.11 Dental cyst   3.12 Internal resorption of the tooth

3.13 Adamantinoma ('ameloblastoma')   3.14 Calcifying epithelial odontogenic tumour   3.15 Giant cell epulis

3.16 Mumps: submandibular salivary gland   3.17 Chronic sialadenitis: parotid gland   3.18 Chronic sialadenitis: parotid gland

3.10 Dentigerous cyst. This form of cyst is frequently found in the region of the third mandibular molar (wisdom tooth) and is derived from odontogenic epithelium. It has a fibrous tissue wall and is lined by stratified squamous epithelium. **3.11 Dental cyst.** This cyst forms in a dental granuloma when trapped epithelial rests proliferate to form a lumen. The result is a fibrous-walled cyst lined by a layer of non-keratinized squamous epithelium (left). There is mild lymphocytic infiltration. **3.12 Internal resorption of the tooth.** The commonest cause of destruction of the dental hard tissues is caries but occasionally chronic inflammation in either the pulp or in the periodontal ligament causes extensive resorption of dentine. Here the enamel has been penetrated and the dentine (right) with its characteristic tubules is being eroded, perhaps by enzymes from the micro-organisms which are growing on the surface of the dentine. A small colony of these is visible at the bottom left corner. The inflammatory exudate (left) is rich in polymorphs. **3.13 Adamantinoma ('ameloblastoma').** This tumour arises from odontogenic epithelium and is ordinarily located in the mandible which it expands. Centrally the lesion consists of cells that resemble the stellate reticulum of the enamel organ. There are also many vacuoles in this region and these sometimes expand to produce a cystic lesion. The central cells are surrounded by and gradually merge with a peripheral layer of compact and deeply basophilic cylindrical cells which bear resemblance to the ameloblasts of the enamel organ. The remaining tissue is fibrous stroma. Though the lesion looks histologically benign it tends to be infiltrative and excision may be difficult or impossible. **3.14 Calcifying epithelial odontogenic tumour.**

There are sheets of closely-packed epithelial cells with basophilic pleomorphic nuclei. There is no evidence of mitotic activity. A dense calcified and laminated body is present (left). This is probably a product of cell degeneration and bodies of this type often first appear as eosinophilic masses which only later calcify and stain blue. **3.15 Giant cell epulis.** This lesion was located in the mandible. The multinucleated giant cells resemble osteoclasts but the stromal cells are relatively mature fibroblasts and have formed a considerable amount of fibrous connective tissue. Though the lesion resembles a giant cell tumour of bone it is reactive and not neoplastic. **3.16 Mumps: submandibular salivary gland.** The glandular tissue has been almost completely destroyed and only a few groups of mucus-secreting cells survive (right). There is a considerable amount of cellular debris scattered among the numerous lymphocytes and plasma cells that have infiltrated the gland. **3.17** and **3.18 Chronic sialadenitis: parotid gland. 3.17** Several lobules of the gland are shown. The acini have disappeared and only ducts remain. There is much fibrous tissue and lymphocytes and plasma cells infiltrate the gland. Some are present within ducts. Vascularity is marked. A calculus was present in the main parotid duct. **3.18** Some normal parotid gland remains (right), the acini being lined with enzyme-secreting (serous) cells. In the chronically inflamed lobule (centre and left) loss of acini is complete and only intercalated ducts remain. There is replacement by fibrous tissue and an inflammatory infiltrate which consists very largely of plasma cells.

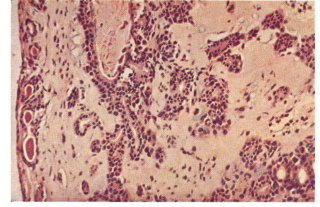

3.19   Pleomorphic adenoma: parotid gland

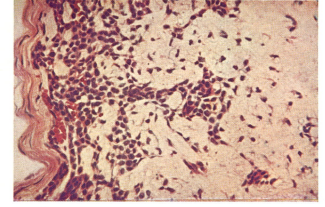

3.20   Pleomorphic adenoma: parotid gland

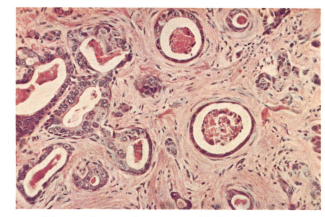

3.21   Primary adenocarcinoma: parotid gland

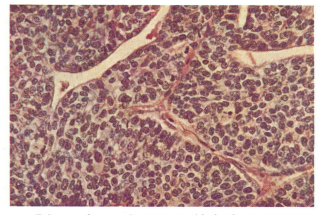

3.22   Primary adenocarcinoma: parotid gland

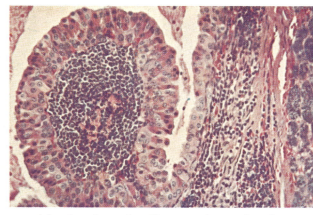

3.23   Adenolymphoma (papillary cystadenoma lymphomatosum): parotid gland

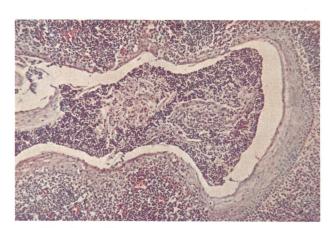

3.24   Chronic tonsillitis

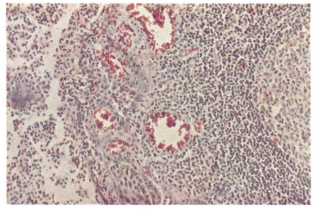

3.25   Chronic tonsillitis

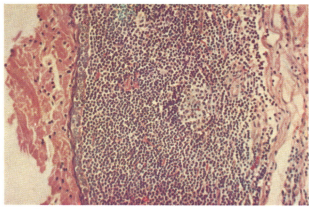

3.26   Lateral cervical branchial cyst

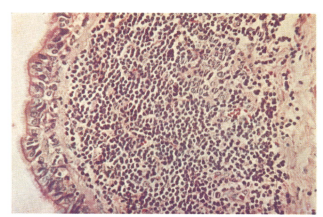

3.27   Lateral cervical branchial cyst

3.19 and **3.20 Pleomorphic adenoma: parotid gland. 3.19** The epithelial cells form acini and duct-like structures. Some of these have a double layer of cells, the outer layer being myoepithelial. The epithelial elements lie in abundant, poorly-vascular myxoid stroma. Also scattered throughout the stroma are cells which cannot be distinguished morphologically from the epithelial cells, some vaguely resembling chondrocytes. **3.20** This is a higher power view to show how the tumour cells grow in irregular cords and sheets which taper off imperceptibly into individual cells which are indistinguishable from the stellate cells of the abundant myxomatous stroma. On the left is the fibrous capsule which did not completely enclose the tumour. **3.21** and **3.22 Primary adenocarcinoma: parotid gland. 3.21** The malignant epithelium forms small clumps and irregular gland-like structures. The cells show considerable pleomorphism, some being small and flattened, others large and columnar. Mitotic figures are not visible here but were present elsewhere. There is abundant fibrous stroma. Some of the debris in the lumen of the malignant gland-like structures is keratinous (right of centre, for example). **3.22** This tumour is relatively undifferentiated and only a few irregular gland-like spaces have formed. The cells have large nuclei with prominent nucleoli and some mitotic activity is evident. The stroma consists only of small blood vessels. **3.23 Adenolymphoma (papillary cystadenoma lymphomatosum): parotid gland.** This is a slow-growing benign tumour, with a well-formed capsule. A portion of normal parotid is present (right), composed of deeply basophilic mucin-secreting

cells. The tumour consists of thick sheets of tall columnar eosinophilic epithelial cells and a lymphoid stroma. The epithelial cells, which are probably derived from ducts, form an irregular cystic space into which a club-shaped mass projects. There is a little mucin in the cystic space. **3.24** and **3.25 Chronic tonsillitis. 3.24** A keratinous plug (centre) is pressing on and apparently causing atrophy of the adjacent epithelial and lymphoid tissues of the tonsil. When many plugs are present they produce an appearance clinically resembling follicular tonsillitis but the inflammatory reaction is lacking. In this instance bacterial colonies are also present along with polymorphs and the tonsil shows increased vascularity. **3.25** This is a higher power view of another crypt of the tonsil shown in 3.24. The lymphoid tissue is hyperplastic and a germinal centre is visible (right). There is hyperaemia, and the capillaries are greatly dilated. The lumen of the crypt contains bacteria (middle left) and inflammatory cells which include polymorphs and lymphocytes. **3.26** and **3.27 Lateral cervical branchial cyst. 3.26** This cyst, which was located near the angle of the mandible and anterior to the sternomastoid muscle, is lined by stratified squamous epithelium that forms abundant keratin (left). Some of the keratinised cells still have nuclei. The wall of the cyst is rich in lymphoid tissue in which there is a germinal follicle. There is a resemblance to thyroglossal duct cyst. **3.27** Less commonly a branchial cyst is lined by columnar epithelium. Here the columnar epithelium is ciliated and resembles respiratory epithelium. As usual the wall of the cyst contains lymphoid tissue.

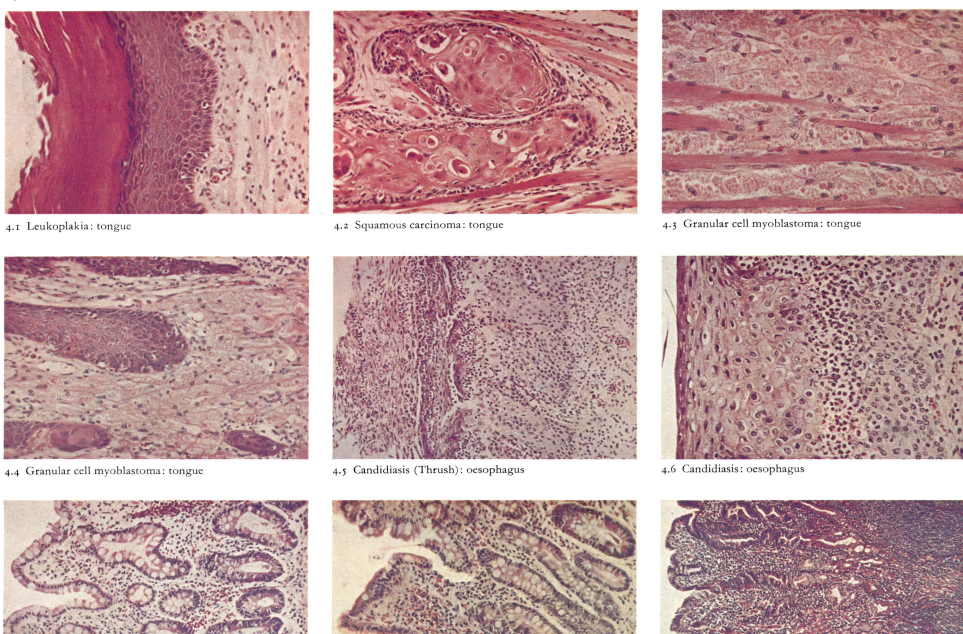

4.1 Leukoplakia: tongue

4.2 Squamous carcinoma: tongue

4.3 Granular cell myoblastoma: tongue

4.4 Granular cell myoblastoma: tongue

4.5 Candidiasis (Thrush): oesophagus

4.6 Candidiasis: oesophagus

4.7 Chronic atrophic gastritis: pernicious anaemia

4.8 Chronic atrophic gastritis: chronic alcoholism

4.9 Ulcer gastritis

4.1 Leukoplakia: tongue. There is pronounced hyperkeratosis and the prickle cell layer (centre) is thickened (acanthosis). In the deepest layers the epithelial cells are pleomorphic, show some loss of polarity and mitotic figures are numerous. Subepithelial inflammatory cell infiltrate is minimal but is sometimes fairly intense. Leukoplakia of the tongue tends to become malignant. **4.2 Squamous carcinoma: tongue.** Long tumour processes are invading the muscle of the tongue. The tumour is well-differentiated and keratinisation is well-developed. There are lymphocytes in the stroma. **4.3 and 4.4 Granular cell myoblastoma: tongue. 4.3** This lesion is usually locally invasive and the large tumour cells are infiltrating between the striated muscle fibres of the tongue which show patchy atrophy. The neoplastic cells have abundant cytoplasm laden with eosinophilic granules, some of which are several microns in diameter. The cells resemble degenerate or embryonic muscle ('myoblastoma') but are derived from Schwann cells. **4.4** The stratified squamous epithelium (left) overlying the tumour cells shows intense hyperplasia, with elongated rete ridges in which there are many mitotic figures. A few of the epithelial processes even look like 'cell-nests'. These epithelial changes (pseudo-epitheliomatous) are apparently induced by the cells of the myoblastoma. **4.5 and 4.6 Candidiasis (Thrush): oesophagus. 4.5** A 'pseudo-membrane' is present (left) on the surface of the stratified squamous epithelium lining the oesophagus. It consists of desquamated epithelial cells and mycelial threads (Candida albicans), just visible as thin filaments at this magnification. The organism has penetrated the superficial layer of the stratified squamous epithelium, which is separating from a relatively unaffected basal layer. A polymorph-rich exudate separates the two layers (centre). The lamina

propria (right) is vascular and infiltrated with lymphocytes and plasma cells. Candida albicans is of low pathogenicity and rarely invades the tissues deeply. Infection is often a consequence of antibiotic therapy. **4.6** This is the same lesion at higher magnification to show the splitting of the stratified squamous epithelium lining the oesophagus into two layers by an acute inflammatory exudate consisting largely of neutrophil polymorphs. The organism growing among these cells is not visible in this preparation but it could be demonstrated by special stains. **4.7 and 4.8 Chronic (atrophic) gastritis. 4.7** The patient suffered from pernicious (Addisonian) anaemia. Parietal and chief (oxyntic) cells have disappeared and instead there is a much thinner structure composed of short glands lined by columnar cells and goblet cells. The tissue resembles atrophic small intestinal mucosa. Plasma cells and lymphocytes are numerous in the interstitial tissue. The muscularis mucosae, just out of the picture on the right, was several times thicker than normal. The small haemorrhages probably occurred while the biopsy specimen was being taken. **4.8** The patient was a chronic alcoholic. The mucosa is similar to 4.7 but the superficial glands are of gastric type and Paneth cells are present at the base of the glands. **4.9 Ulcer gastritis.** This is the gastric mucosa in the vicinity of a chronic peptic ulcer. The most notable feature is the intense diffuse infiltration by chronic inflammatory cells including lymphoid follicles (top right). The normal surface epithelium consists of a regular line of columnar mucin-secreting cells but here it has been replaced by an irregular line of pleomorphic, basophilic cells and goblet cells. Similar cells line the glands. Care must be taken not to mistake the irregular epithelium adjacent to an ulcer for carcinoma.

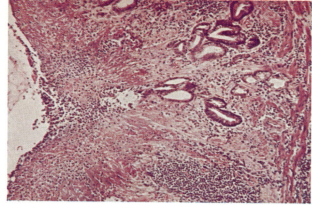

4.10 Acute erosion: stomach

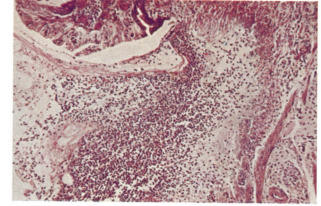

4.11 Acute ulcer: stomach

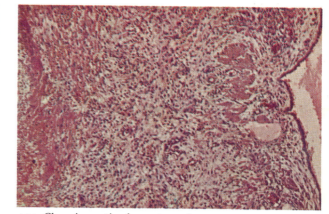

4.12 Chronic peptic ulcer: stomach

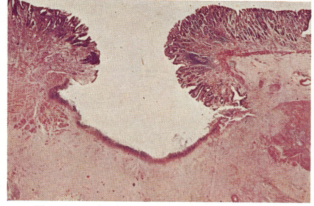

4.13 Chronic peptic ulcer: stomach

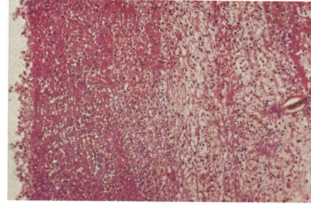

4.14 Chronic peptic ulcer: stomach

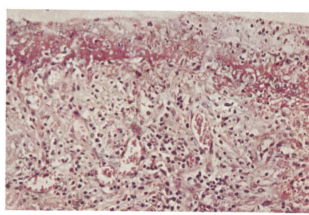

4.15 Chronic peptic ulcer: stomach

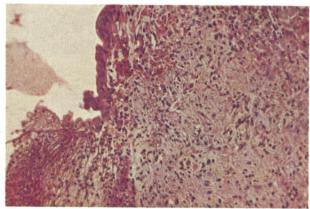

4.16 Chronic peptic ulcer: stomach

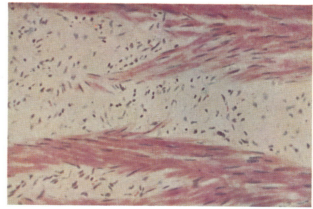

4.17 Primary scirrhous carcinoma: stomach

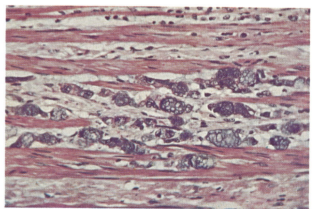

4.18 Primary adenocarcinoma: stomach

4.10 Acute erosion: stomach. The surface epithelium has disappeared and the superficial half of the mucosa (left) is necrotic, being deeply eosinophilic and containing only nuclear fragments. The lymphoid tissue (below) is a normal feature. The muscularis mucosae is on the right. **4.11 Acute ulcer: stomach.** This is an early phase in its formation. The whole thickness of the mucosa is necrotic and the muscularis mucosae (right) has been breached. Nuclear debris is scattered throughout the necrotic tissue and some fragments of gastric epithelium are visible (top left). When the necrotic tissue sloughs an acute ulcer will result. Acute ulcers are often multiple, and are found in uraemia, after extensive burns, and in association with hypothalamic lesions. Many are of unknown aetiology. **4.12–4.16 Chronic peptic ulcer: stomach. 4.12** This is the subserosa. The ulcer has penetrated through almost the whole thickness of the stomach wall and its necrotic floor is just visible on the left. A vigorous inflammatory reaction in the subserosa has produced a considerable quantity of granulation tissue and young connective tissue in which chronic inflammatory cells are plentiful (centre). A little sero-fibrinous exudate covers the hyperplastic serosal cells (right). A fragment of smooth muscle survives in this tissue. **4.13** The ulcer has destroyed the muscle coats of the stomach, which are visible on the right and left. The floor of the ulcer consists of necrotic debris and dense fibrous tissue. The gastric epithelium is hyperplastic and tends to overhang the crater but it is not heaped-up. Its altered histological appearance may be mistaken for malignant change. **4.14** This is the floor of an active ulcer. It is covered with fibrinous exudate and necrotic cells. A 'foreign body' is present (right centre) within the fibrin network. **4.15** Healing is taking place. The fibrin and necrotic debris have been removed and the floor of the ulcer consists of healthy granulation tissue. **4.16** This is the edge of an ulcer. The crater has filled with young connective tissue (right), and although a layer of fibrin and necrotic debris remains on the surface (below left), epithelial cells are beginning to migrate from the adjacent mucosa. The migrating cells are a single layer of cuboidal cells (above left). **4.17 Primary scirrhous carcinoma: stomach.** The tumour was a diffuse or spreading type of lesion which formed a scirrhous plaque but did not project into the lumen. This is part of the greatly thickened muscle coat involved in the plaque. The muscle fibres are separated by connective tissue throughout which are scattered small dark-staining cells. These are undifferentiated carcinoma cells and are easily overlooked. Sometimes the malignant cells can be identified by staining the mucin in their cytoplasm. The connective tissue is the tumour stroma and when this type of tumour is extensive it forms a 'leather-bottle' stomach (linitis plastica). **4.18 Primary adenocarcinoma: stomach.** The tumour formed a large ulcer with an elevated irregular border. This shows the adjacent muscle coat. It is extensively invaded by tumour cells which contain deeply basophilic mucin, in amounts sufficients to obscure the cell nuclei. Some fibrous stroma has formed.

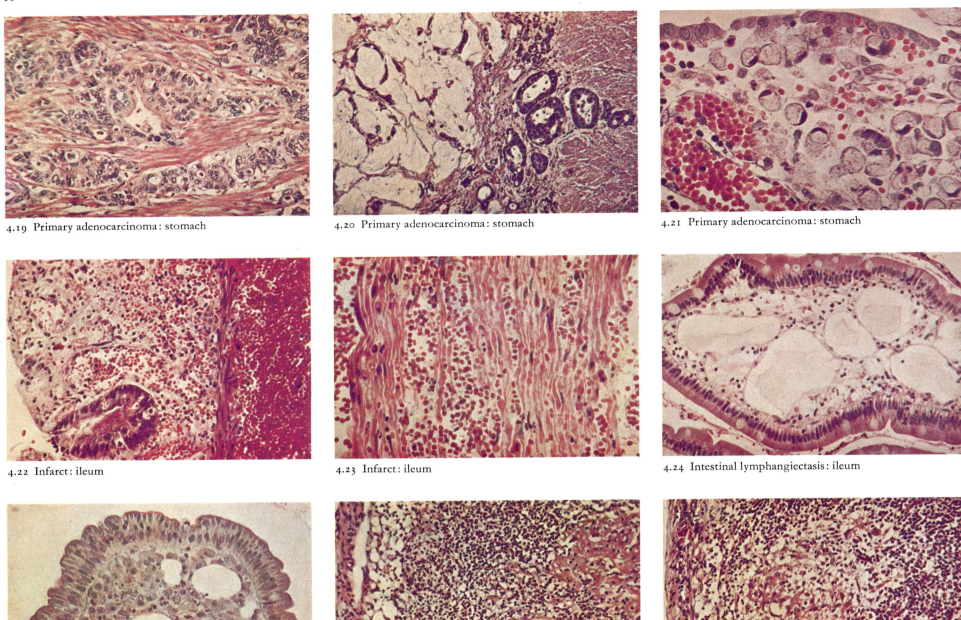

4.19 Primary adenocarcinoma: stomach

4.20 Primary adenocarcinoma: stomach

4.21 Primary adenocarcinoma: stomach

4.22 Infarct: ileum

4.23 Infarct: ileum

4.24 Intestinal lymphangiectasis: ileum

4.25 Intestinal lipodystrophy (Whipple's disease): jejunum

4.26 Intestinal lipodystrophy: lymph node

4.27 Intestinal lipodystrophy: lymph node

4.19–4.21 Primary adenocarcinoma: stomach. 4.19 This lesion is similar to 4.18 but mucin secretion is not a feature. The cells invading and destroying the muscle coats are large and pleomorphic and form imperfect acini. **4.20** This is a mucoid (colloid) carcinoma. The malignant epithelial cells, in cords and irregular acini, are floating in large quantities of mucin (left) which they have secreted. The tumour cells have large basophilic nuclei. Invasion of the muscle coats (right) is beginning. **4.21** This is the serosal surface. The serosal cells (top) are unusually prominent and many mucin-laden tumour cells are lying in the subserosa. The neoplastic cells contain so much mucin in their cytoplasm that the nucleus of each cell has been pushed to the side to produce a 'signet-ring' shape. The cells can detach themselves and spread throughout the peritoneal cavity to produce peritoneal carcinomatosis. Gastric carcinomas also spread readily by the portal vein to the liver. **4.22** and **4.23 Infarct: ileum.** The lesion followed mesenteric vein thrombosis. The bowel was greatly swollen and deep purple. **4.22** The villous structure has been lost and only a crypt (bottom left) remains, lined by cells which show altered nuclear staining and are probably necrotic. The capillaries are greatly distended and there is extensive haemorrhage (right) deep to the muscularis mucosae. **4.23** The fibres of the muscle coats are necrotic. They have partly or entirely lost their nuclear staining and are very distorted. Haemorrhage is very extensive. **4.24 Intestinal lymphangiectasis: ileum.** This patient had longstanding and widespread obstruction of lymphatic channels. The lacteals were distended with lipid and there was chylous ascites. In this section the dilated lacteals fill the core of the villus. There is no inflammatory or fibrotic reaction round them, and the intestinal epithelium appears normal. **4.25–4.27 Intestinal lipodystrophy (Whipple's disease).** In this rare condition fat absorption is disturbed. **4.25** The columnar epithelial cells of the jejunum are normal but the core of the villus is packed with large macrophages which have abundant rather greyish 'frosted-glass' cytoplasm. The material in the cytoplasm responsible for this colour often gives positive reactions for both polysaccharide and lipid. There are a few scattered polymorphs. The spaces are dilated lymphatic channels (lacteals) which have lost their lipid contents during processing of the tissues. Electron microscopy showed many bacillus-like bodies lying between the macrophages. **4.26** The peripheral sinus (left) of this mesenteric lymph node is distended with vacuoles which contained lipo-polysaccharide. Deeper in the node (right) there is an eosinophilic area of sclerosis. This second lesion is not specific and is found in chronic lymphadenitis. **4.27** A much more characteristic granulomatous focus (centre) is present, however, in the subcapsular region of this node. Macrophages are clustered round vacuoles that contained lipo-polysaccharide. The macrophages vaguely resemble epithelioid cells and the focus is reminiscent of a tubercle follicle.

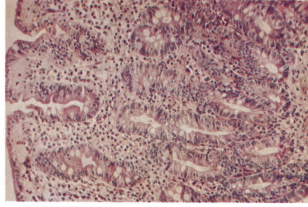

4.28 Idiopathic steatorrhoea: jejunum

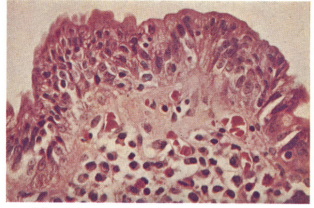

4.29 Idiopathic steatorrhoea: jejunum

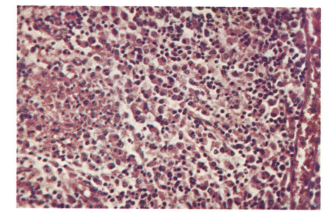

4.30 Typhoid fever: ileum

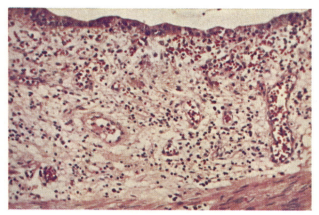

4.31 Healed ulcer (regional enteritis): ileum

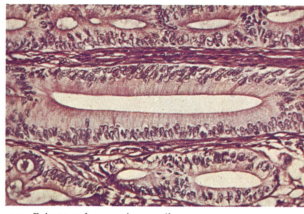

4.32 Primary adenocarcinoma: ileum

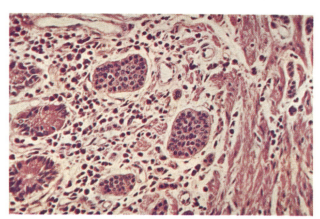

4.33 Argentaffin carcinoma (carcinoid tumour): caecum

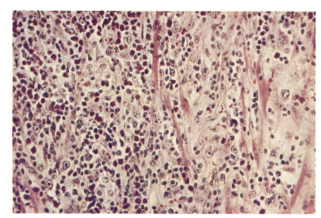

4.34 Hodgkin's disease (mixed cell type): ileum

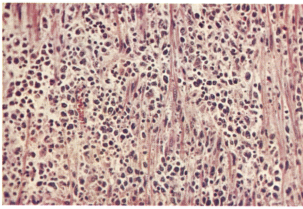

4.35 Reticulum cell sarcoma: ileum

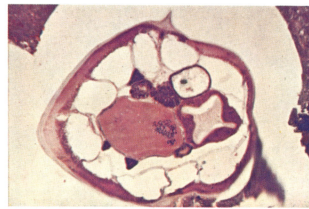

4.36 Threadworm (Pinworm): appendix

4.28 and **4.29 Idiopathic steatorrhoea: jejunum. 4.28** The mucosa is thinner than normal and the tall villi of the normal gut have been replaced by very short flat structures (left). Paradoxically however, the crypts (middle and right) are considerably longer than normal. The epithelial cells lining the crypts and glands are somewhat pleomorphic. The cells covering the surface are flat and degenerate-looking and rest upon a thick hyalinised basement membrane. Plasma cells and lymphocytes are scattered throughout the mucosa. **4.29** This shows in more detail the great thickening of the epithelial basement membrane that often occurs. The new material is hyaline and amorphous and it surrounds the capillaries. There are many plasma cells in the lamina propria. The normal tall columnar epithelial cells have been replaced by pleomorphic cells. **4.30 Typhoid fever: ileum.** This is a lymphoid (Peyer's) patch in the terminal ileum. It is hyperaemic and heavily infiltrated with mononuclear inflammatory cells. These are nearly all macrophages, though scattered plasma cells and lymphocytes are also present. The patient had been ill for about 10 days and necrotic foci are now appearing (left of centre). A Gram stain would reveal large numbers of typhoid bacilli. During recovery the necrotic cells are phagocytosed and epithelium quickly grows over the ulcerated area, so that fibrosis is minimal. **4.31 Healed ulcer (regional enteritis).** The patient suffered from regional enteritis (Crohn's disease) and this shows a part of the ileal mucosa that was previously ulcerated. A single layer of cuboidal or low columnar epithelial cells covers a layer of mature granulation tissue which in turn rests upon the circular muscle coat (bottom) of the intestine. The new epithelium is incapable of restoring the normal villus structure. **4.32 Primary adenocarcinoma: ileum.** This is the muscle coat. It has been replaced at this point by a particularly well-differentiated adenocarcinoma, the cells

of which closely resemble those of normal small intestine. They are tall and columnar, their nuclei are basal in position, a brush border is present, and they form elongated very regular glands. Primary carcinomas of the small intestine are comparatively rare and a secondary growth from the colon can simulate the condition. **4.33 Argentaffin carcinoma (carcinoid tumour).** The tumour was a yellow nodule in the wall of the caecum. Compact solid groups of characteristic cells (centre) are present in the mucosa beneath the glands (left) of the gut and smaller groups are also invading the muscle coats (right). The cells are of uniform type and there are no mitoses. The cells rarely secrete mucin or form glands. They produce serotonin (5-hydroxytryptamine) and the presence of large deposits of tumour, usually in the liver, leads to the characteristic clinical syndrome of pulmonary stenosis, tricuspid incompetence, vasomotor symptoms, bronchial obstruction and an unusual type of cyanosis. The cells lying between the tumour cell clumps and the intestinal glands are eosinophil leucocytes. **4.34 Hodgkin's disease (mixed cell type): ileum.** The muscle coats are almost destroyed by tumour which consists very largely of malignant reticulum cells. Characteristically large numbers of eosinophil leucocytes are present. There were deposits of Hodgkin's tissue in other organs. **4.35 Reticulum cell sarcoma: ileum.** Malignant and highly pleomorphic reticulum cells have almost replaced the muscle coats. **4.36 Threadworm (Pinworm): appendix.** This is a cross-section of a threadworm (Enterobius vermicularis) lying in the lumen of the appendix. Sometimes a worm penetrates into the submucosa, dies and excites a granulomatous reaction, with epithelioid cells, lymphocytes and eosinophils surrounding necrotic remnants of the parasite.

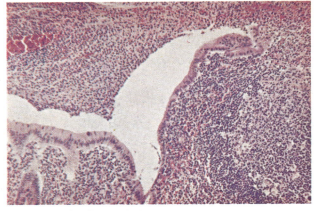

4.37 Acute focal appendicitis

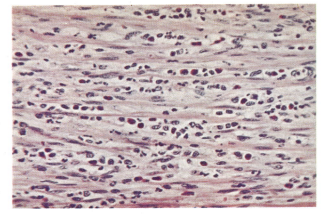

4.38 Acute diffuse suppurative appendicitis

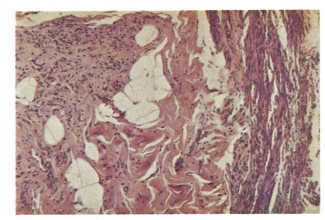

4.39 Chronic obliterative appendicitis

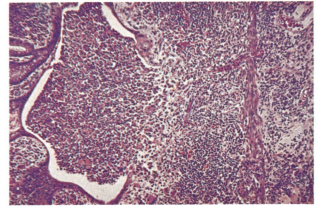

4.40 Regional enteritis (Crohn's disease)

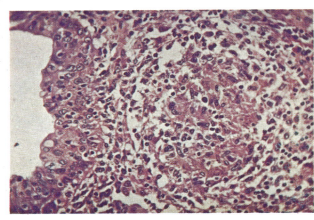

4.41 Regional enteritis

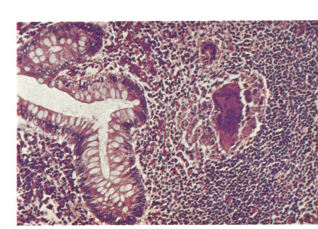

4.42 Regional enteritis

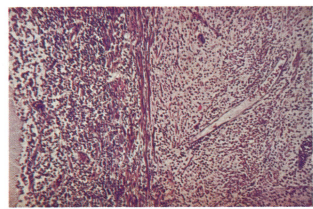

4.43 Regional enteritis

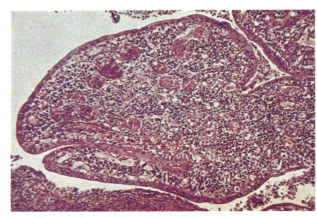

4.44 Regional enteritis

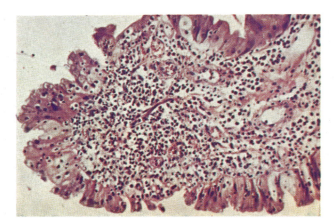

4.45 Regional enteritis

4.37 Acute focal appendicitis. This is near the tip of the organ. The lumen is filled with pus (top left) which contains many red cells. The mucosa (bottom) is infiltrated with polymorphs and the epithelium is ulcerated (top right). The lymphoid follicle (right) has a prominent germinal centre but is not otherwise noteworthy. **4.38 Acute diffuse suppurative appendicitis.** This is the muscle coat. The fibres are separated by inflammatory exudate containing many polymorphs. There are also a number of macrophages. The high proportion of eosinophils suggests that the lesion had been present for several days. **4.39 Chronic obliterative appendicitis.** The muscle coats are visible on the right. There is no mucosa and the lumen (left) has been completely obliterated by fibrous tissue and fat. These changes may be the result of previous inflammatory episodes though some believe that they are involutionary. **4.40–4.45 Regional enteritis (Crohn's disease). 4.40** A mass of inflammatory cells has collected deep to the intestinal glands (left) to form a crypt abscess. The cells are mainly polymorphs but macrophages and occasional giant cells are present in the deeper part of the abscess. Epithelial cells partly line the abscess cavity. The abscess may have started in the gland crypt or it may have ruptured into it. Chronic inflammatory cells are very numerous on both sides of the muscularis mucosae (right) which is intact. Lesions similar to this are seen in ulcerative colitis and histological separation of the two conditions is often impossible. However Crohn's disease is generally distinguished on the basis of the following features: the deep fissures, extending into the muscle coats or to the serosa; severe oedema in the submucosa and subserosa; and sarcoid granulomas in the gut and lymph nodes. **4.41** This

patient had lesions which extended from the ileum to the anus. In this section of the anal mucosa a follicular collection of epithelioid cells is present beneath the stratified squamous epithelium (left). There is no caseation in the follicle which resembles a sarcoid granuloma and tubercle bacilli could not be demonstrated. There are a few lymphocytes round the granuloma but no attempt at fibrotic repair. Lymphocytes and polymorphs are migrating through the epithelium. **4.42** This is a similar lesion in the colon. A small follicular collection of epithelioid cells (right of centre) and multinucleated giant cells lies in the lymphoid tissue (right) of the hyperaemic lamina propria. The overlying mucus-secreting colonic gland (left) is intact but it is surrounded by plasma cells. **4.43** There has been complete destruction of the mucosa and the muscle coats are reduced to a few thin fibres (centre). The gut is lined by granulation tissue (left) rich in chronic inflammatory cells. Similar tissue, but more fibrous, forms a layer on the serosa (right). **4.44** The mucosa of the terminal ileum has been replaced by a polypoid mass of granulation tissue rich in capillaries and chronic inflammatory cells. The 'polyp' here is covered by a single layer of large cuboidal epithelial cells. A considerable amount of fibrin-rich exudate (bottom) lies between the polypoid masses. **4.45** This is a similar lesion in the colon. The mucosa has been raised in polypoid fashion and the granulation tissue that forms the core of this polyp is heavily infiltrated with inflammatory cells which are a mixture of polymorphs and plasma cells. Many polymorphs are migrating through the epithelium, the cells of which though mostly columnar show considerable diversity of structure. Some are mucin-secreting. They form an incomplete covering to the polyp.

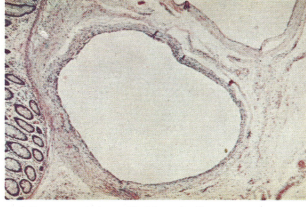

4.46 Pneumatosis (cystoides) intestinalis

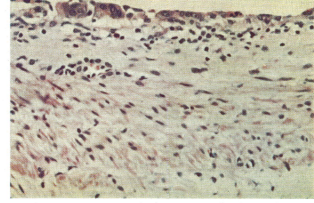

4.47 Pneumatosis intestinalis

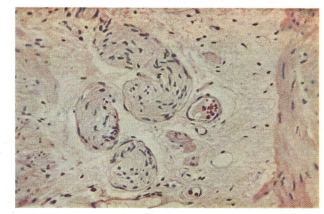

4.48 Primary megacolon (Hirschsprung's disease)

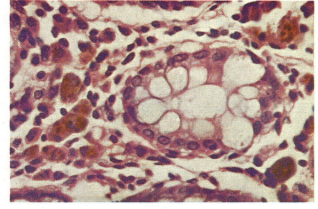

4.49 Melanosis coli

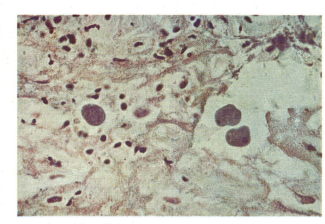

4.50 Amoebic colitis

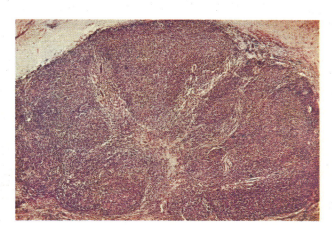

4.51 Benign lymphoid growth: rectum

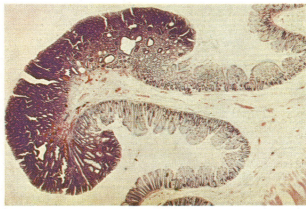

4.52 Adenomatous polyp (papilloma): colon

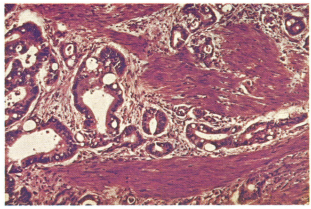

4.53 Primary adenocarcinoma: colon

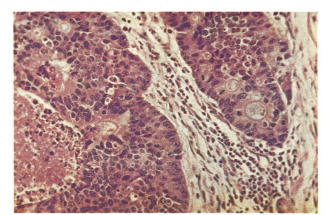

4.54 Primary adenocarcinoma: colon

4.46 and **4.47 Pneumatosis (cystoides) intestinalis.** This condition usually affects the small intestine but here the lesion is in the colon. There are large numbers of gas-filled cysts in the submucosa. The aetiology is unknown but it may be that gas from the lumen enters and distends the lymphatics. The cysts may produce intestinal obstruction. **4.46** One of the smaller cysts is shown (centre) and part of a larger one at the top right. Each cyst has a thin wall of fibromuscular tissue. The colonic mucosa and muscularis muscosae are on the left. **4.47** This is a higher power view of the cyst wall. There is a granulomatous reaction and phagocytes (top), many multinucleated, line the gas-filled spaces. A thin layer of fibromuscular tissue also forms part of the wall. **4.48 Primary megacolon (Hirschsprung's disease).** This is the colon distal to the dilated part. In the loose connective tissues between the inner (left) and outer (right) muscle coats of the colon lies the myenteric nerve plexus (centre). Medullated nerve fibres are present but ganglion cells (parasympathetic) are lacking. Consequently the bowel was unable to relax and mechanical obstruction resulted. Removal of the affected part of the colon is curative if performed sufficiently early. It should be noted that ganglion cells are present in the dilated gut. **4.49 Melanosis coli.** The colonic mucosa was brownish-black in appearance. Many pigment-laden macrophages are lying in the tissues around the mucin-secreting colonic glands. The pigment is not melanin but lipofuscin. It may be formed in situ from absorbed products of protein decomposition such as tryptophane. The condition has no clinical significance. **4.50 Amoebic colitis.** This is the submucosa of the caecum. Three vegetative (trophozoite) forms of Entamoeba histolytica are present. The parasites have produced coagulative necrosis of the surround-

ing tissues but have evoked almost no cellular reaction. Each amoeba has abundant refractile, vacuolated cytoplasm but none contains erythrocytes. The fact that E. histolytica usually contains ingested red cells and has only one to four nuclei helps to distinguish it from the non-pathogenic E. coli. **4.51 Benign lymphoid growth: rectum.** The lesion presented as a polyp in the rectum. A well-demarcated ovoid mass of lymphoid tissue lies in the submucosa. There is a vaguely follicular pattern but higher power examination shows that the lymphoid cells are mature. The lesion is probably hamartomatous. **4.52 Adenomatous polyp (papilloma): colon.** This lesion has a pedicle of delicate connective tissue covered with normal mucin-secreting colonic mucosa. However the top of the polyp is covered with a very thick layer of basophilic cells which form very irregular glands and have mostly lost their mucin-secreting capabilities. Though high-power examination showed nuclear pleomorphism and occasional mitotic activity with a poorly-formed and ill-defined basement membrane, no definite invasion of the connective tissue of the stalk could be detected and malignant change had probably not yet supervened. **4.53** and **4.54 Primary adenocarcinoma: colon. 4.53** The tumour consists of irregular poorly-formed acini. It is invading the muscle coats. **4.54** The tumour has penetrated to the pericolic tissues. Its cells are poorly differentiated and have largely lost their capacity for secreting mucin and even for forming gland-like structures. Mitoses are numerous and there is extensive necrosis (left). Lymphocytes are present around the growing edge of the neoplasm (bottom right). Carcinomas of the colon spread not only by lymphatics but also readily by the portal vein to the liver.

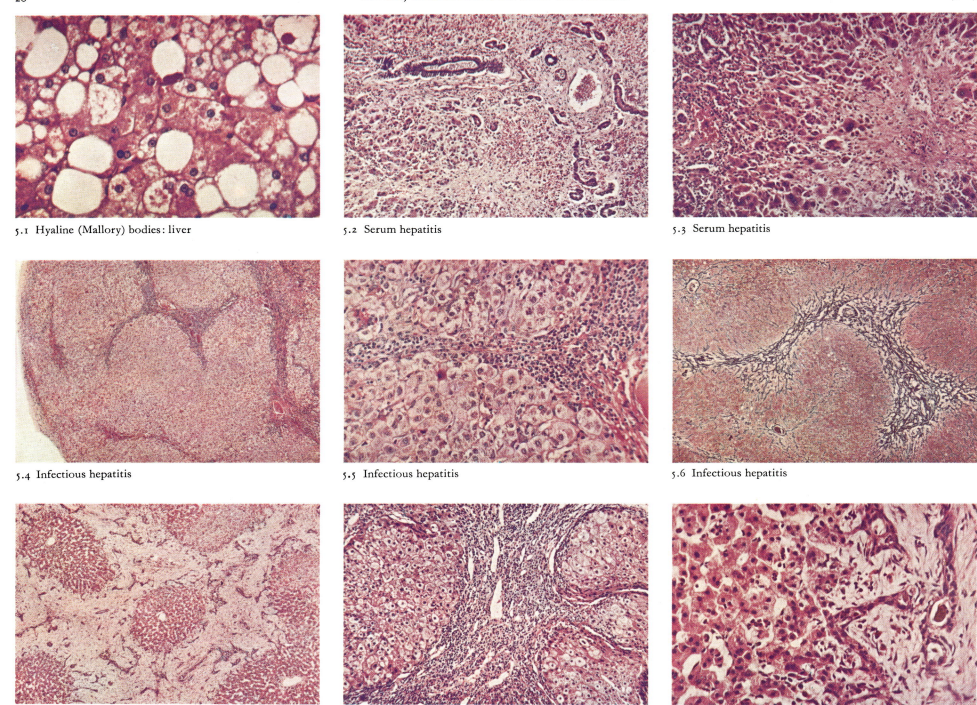

5.1 Hyaline (Mallory) bodies: liver

5.2 Serum hepatitis

5.3 Serum hepatitis

5.4 Infectious hepatitis

5.5 Infectious hepatitis

5.6 Infectious hepatitis

5.7 Portal cirrhosis

5.8 Portal cirrhosis

5.9 Portal cirrhosis

5.1 Hyaline (Mallory) bodies: liver. This is part of a regeneration nodule in a cirrhotic liver. Many of the parenchymal cells are full of fat and in several there are also dense red spherical bodies (top right for example). Similar eosinophilic masses are sometimes seen in non-alcoholic portal cirrhosis and in livers damaged experimentally. The lesion is an example of focal cytoplasmic degeneration and electron microscopy shows that the bodies contain a variety of cytoplasmic organelles such as mitochondria and lysosomes. **5.2** and **5.3 Serum hepatitis. 5.2** The parenchymal cells in the vicinity of the portal vein (right) have disappeared and the bile-ducts are correspondingly prominent. The sinusoids are distended and there is haemorrhage. The remaining liver cells (bottom left) look unhealthy. **5.3** This shows in more detail the centrilobular necrosis (right) and the abnormal appearance of the surviving liver cells: their size and shape vary greatly, and many are binucleate. Small necrotic bile-laden cells are also present. Lymphocytic infiltration is intense. There is considerable fibrous tissue formation around the portal tract (right). **5.4–5.6 Infectious hepatitis.** The patient had infectious hepatitis eight months prior to biopsy. **5.4** Fibrous tissue heavily infiltrated with lymphocytes has formed in and around the portal tracts. It is also tending to link the portal tracts and divide the liver into irregular nodules. This 'pre-cirrhotic' change has been brought about by persistent infection and continued destruction of parenchymal cells by the virus. **5.5** is a higher power view of part of 5.4. The fibrous tissue that has formed round the portal vein (right) runs (left) to join a neighbouring portal tract. It is heavily infiltrated with lymphocytes. Necrotic liver cells occur singly or in small groups (left of centre, for example). **5.6** A silver stain for reticulin has been used to demonstrate

more clearly the degree of fibrosis. It shows dark-staining fibres surrounding and linking the portal tracts. Fibrosis of this degree may still be reversible. The method also makes visible the delicate reticulin network of the normal parts of the liver. **5.7–5.9 Portal cirrhosis.** Cirrhosis, according to Sherlock, should be applied only to livers showing a characteristic pattern of hepatic cell necrosis, nodular regeneration, variable connective tissue proliferation and a disturbed hepatic architecture. It should not be used for fibrosis without distortion of the lobular architecture. This definition excludes lesions like those in 5.4 to 5.6, where there is no nodular regeneration. **5.7** The liver cells round the central vein are intact but the periportal cells have been replaced by mature fibrous tissue in which numerous bile ducts are visible. The distribution of the fibrous tissue is unusually regular in this case so that the nodules of parenchymal cells are of uniform size. Nevertheless there is evidence of regeneration in the nodules and in one (top left) the centrilobular vein is markedly eccentric. **5.8** In this case the scarring was much less regular and divides the liver into regeneration nodules that vary greatly in size, some being more than 5 mm. in diameter. Four of the smaller nodules are seen here. Running between them are broad bands of fibrous tissue in which there are many lymphocytes and plasma cells. **5.9** This is the edge of a regeneration nodule. There is biliary stasis and inspissated bile fills the lumen of the small bile-duct lying in the dense fibrous tissue (right). Several small groups of necrotic liver cells are being digested by polymorphs (below and left of centre, for example) and macrophages laden with bile pigment are present near the bile-duct. These appearances are rarely seen even in advanced portal cirrhosis and are more typical of extrahepatic biliary obstruction.

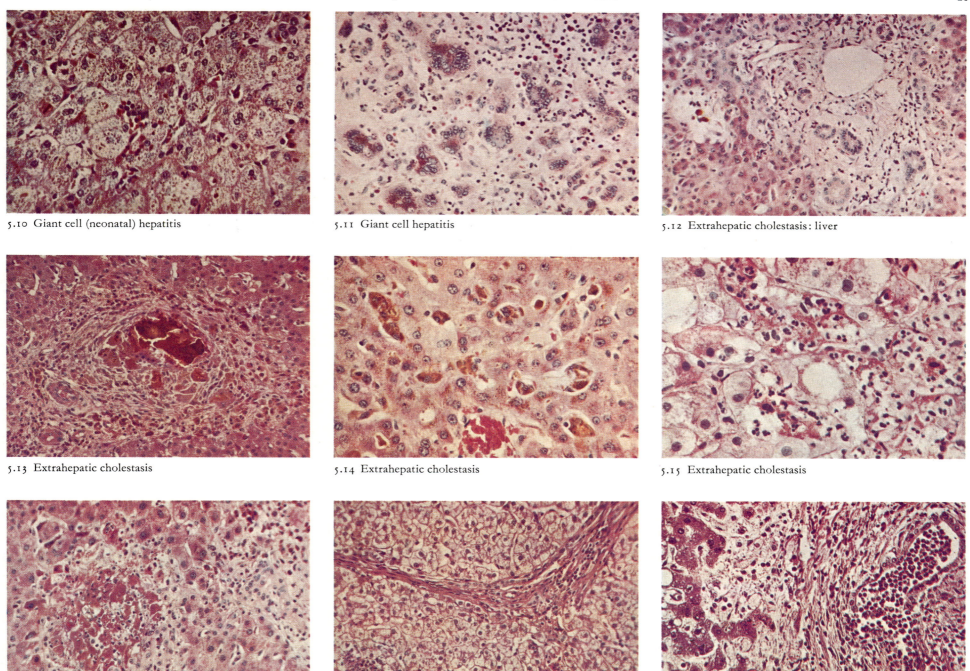

5.10 Giant cell (neonatal) hepatitis

5.11 Giant cell hepatitis

5.12 Extrahepatic cholestasis: liver

5.13 Extrahepatic cholestasis

5.14 Extrahepatic cholestasis

5.15 Extrahepatic cholestasis

5.16 Extrahepatic cholestasis

5.17 Extrahepatic cholestasis

5.18 Suppurative cholangitis

5.10 and **5.11 Giant cell (neonatal) hepatitis.** This is a form of viral hepatitis that is transmitted to the fetus *in utero*. It may be fully developed at birth. **5.10** The liver cells are very large and some are binucleate. Bile pigment is present within them and pigment fills many canaliculi. Glycogen is responsible for the pale granular appearance of the cytoplasm. The Kupffer cells are prominent. Lymphocytic infiltration is comparatively slight. **5.11** There is complete disorganisation of structure and the surviving liver cells are large, multinucleate and laden with bile pigment. The stroma is oedematous and infiltrated with lymphocytes and eosinophils. **5.12–5.17 Extrahepatic cholestasis: liver.** In these cases, the common bile duct was obstructed by a calculus. **5.12** This is a portal tract and the striking feature is the amount of inflammatory oedema. This is causing wide separation of the various elements, the bileducts, the hepatic artery and the portal vein, but leucocytic infiltration is relatively slight. Biliary stasis is evident (left) and some parenchymal cells are necrotic. **5.13** In the centre is a mass of concentrated bile pigment surrounded by pigment-laden phagocytes and degenerating liver cells (bile lake). There is early fibrous tissue formation around it. A branch of the hepatic artery is visible (bottom left). **5.14** The canaliculi are filled with bile (bile thrombi) and bile pigment is also present within liver cells

and Kupffer cells. The vessel at the bottom is the central (hepatic) vein. **5.15** There is widespread necrosis of liver cells and polymorphs are removing the dead cells. Many of the other liver cells are degenerate and vacuolated. **5.16** This is a larger group of necrotic parenchymal cells (left). The dead cells are being digested and removed by phagocytes. Isolated necrotic cells are also visible (top left, for example). Bile-laden macrophages are gathered (top right) on the fringe of the oedematous portal tract (right). **5.17** The common bile duct had been obstructed for several months and there is now definite fibrosis, with fibrous tissue bands running between the portal tracts. There is some infiltration of the fibrous tissue by lymphocytes. A small group of necrotic liver cells is being engulfed by polymorphs (bottom left). In some cases of obstructive jaundice, the extrahepatic ducts are patent and the obstruction to bile flow is confined to the intrahepatic cholangioles or to the liver cells themselves. **5.18 Suppurative cholangitis.** The lumen of the small intrahepatic bile-duct (right) is full of pus and its epithelial lining has broken down. Around the duct there is inflammatory oedema, cellular infiltration and fibrosis. The bile canaliculi are distended with bile and the liver cells show fatty change.

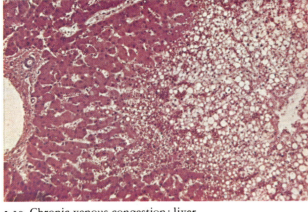

5.19 Chronic venous congestion: liver

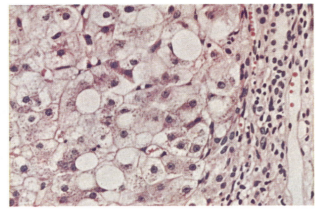

5.20 Fatty change: liver

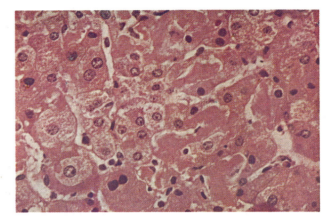

5.21 Amyloid: liver

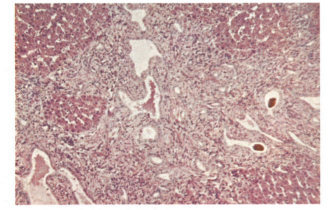

5.22 Congenital hepatic fibrosis

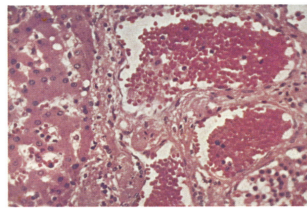

5.23 Cavernous haemangioma: liver

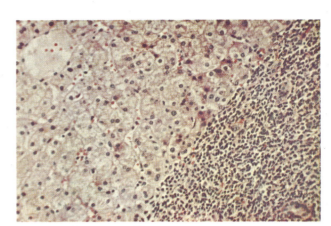

5.24 Lymphosarcoma: liver

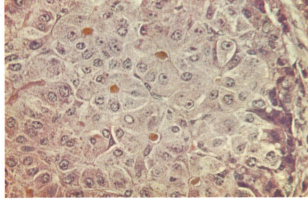

5.25 Primary carcinoma: liver

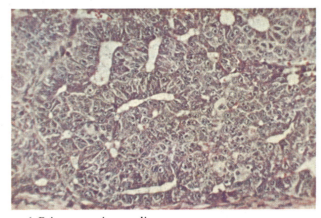

5.26 Primary carcinoma: liver

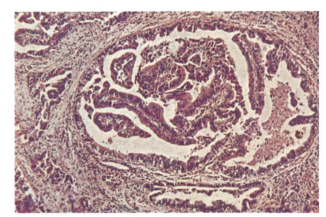

5.27 Primary carcinoma: bile duct

5.19 Chronic venous congestion: liver. The liver cells at the periphery of the lobule (left) look normal but in the centrilobular zone (right) the liver cells are full of fat and many are atrophic. The sinusoids are very distended. In more severe cases many cells disappear and fibrous tissue apparently increases. Macroscopically the contrast between the brown colour of the peripheral cells and the yellow colour of the fatty central cells is one way that the 'nutmeg' pattern characteristic of chronic passive congestion is produced. In the portal tract (left) a branch of the portal vein and a small bile duct are visible. **5.20 Fatty change: liver.** Though many of the liver cells are healthy, the cytoplasm appearing granular from the abundant glycogen present, other cells contain large droplets of fat. These appear as clear vacuoles, the fat having dissolved during processing of the tissue. This is part of a cirrhotic liver and the fibrous tissue in the portal tract (right) is infiltrated with lymphocytes. **5.21 Amyloid: liver.** The parenchymal cells are separated from the sinusoids by a dense pink amorphous deposit of amyloid. Some of the liver cells are atrophic, from pressure atrophy and ischaemia. The Kupffer cells are easily recognised. This is secondary amyloidosis, the patient suffering from rheumatoid arthritis. **5.22 Congenital hepatic fibrosis.** The patient was aged 15 and had polycystic kidneys. The liver was enlarged but not noticeably polycystic and there was portal hypertension. This biopsy shows abundant cellular fibrous tissue in which there are numerous dilated bile-ducts, some containing dense plugs of bile (middle right). The fibrous tissue divides the parenchymal cells into nodules (a small one is visible middle left). **5.23 Cavernous haemangioma: liver.** This was a dark red wedge-shaped lesion situated beneath the capsule of the liver. It consists of large venous chan-

nels with thick fibrous walls and is probably hamartomatous in nature. **5.24 Lymphosarcoma: liver.** The neoplastic cells are small mature lymphocytes and they have heavily infiltrated the portal zone (right). The deposit is well demarcated and the centrilobular zone (top left) is free. Isolated parenchymal cells are degenerating and their cytoplasm is dense and hyaline. A similar appearance is found in chronic lymphocytic leukaemia. A small bile-duct is visible (bottom right). **5.25 and 5.26 Primary carcinoma: liver. 5.25** This is a hepatocarcinoma (hepatoma), the tumour cells being well-differentiated and resembling liver cells. A plug of bile pigment is present at the centre of several clusters of cells. At the periphery of the tumour nodule (right) the cells are compressed and degenerate. Hepatocarcinoma is sometimes associated with portal cirrhosis. It is then usually widespread throughout the liver and perhaps of multicentric origin. **5.26** This is cholangiocarcinoma, the tumour resembling bile duct epithelium and forming crude tubules and ducts. It is similar to carcinoma of the extrahepatic ducts. In this example the large size of the nucleoli in the tumour cells is a feature but mitotic activity was moderate throughout the tumour. **5.27 Primary carcinoma: bile duct.** The tumour was a small mass near the ampulla of Vater. It is a papilliferous adenocarcinoma. The tall columnar epithelium forms small and large glands, some containing necrotic cellular debris, and into these long finger-like processes are growing. The stroma is abundant and fibrous and it is heavily infiltrated with lymphocytes. Carcinomas of the bile ducts are sometimes remarkably well-differentiated and composed of small mature-looking ducts.

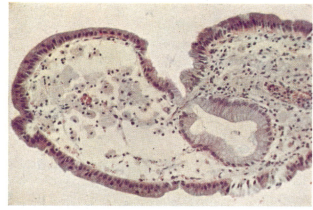

5.28 Cholesterolosis ('strawberry gallbladder')

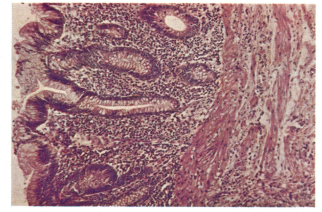

5.29 Chronic cholecystitis

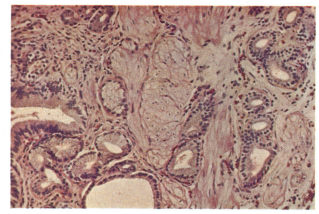

5.30 Chronic cholecystitis

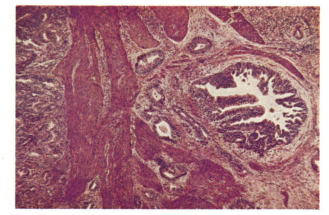

5.31 Primary carcinoma: gallbladder

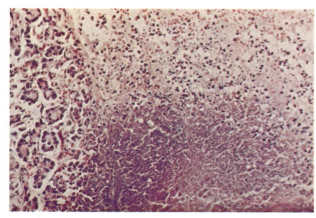

5.32 Acute haemorrhagic pancreatitis

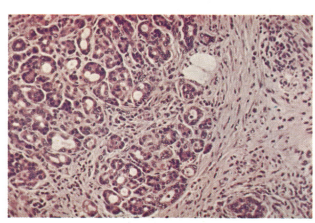

5.33 Diffuse chronic sclerosing pancreatitis

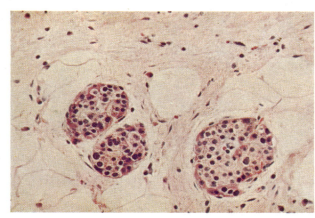

5.34 Atrophy: pancreas

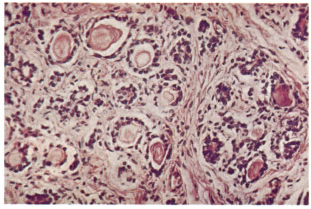

5.35 Mucoviscidosis (fibrocystic disease): pancreas

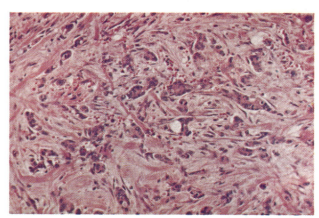

5.36 Primary carcinoma: pancreas

5.28 Cholesterolosis ('strawberry gallbladder'). A bright yellow deposit was present in the mucosal folds. This is a cross-section of one of the affected folds and it shows an infiltrate of macrophages with a foamy or frosted-glass (lipid-laden) cytoplasm. It is the lipid in these cells that gives the mucosal streaks their yellow colour. Cholesterolosis precedes formation of gallstones and both are often present together. **5.29** and **5.30 Chronic cholecystitis.** The gallbladder was small and contained many 'mixed' gall-stones. **5.29** The mucosa (left) is thick and lacks the normal folds. It is very heavily infiltrated with inflammatory cells, lymphocytes, plasma cells and eosinophils. The muscle coat is markedly hypertrophied but chronic inflammatory cells are relatively few and fibrosis is slight. **5.30** The mucosal epithelium has proliferated and grown through the fibrosed and hypertrophied muscle coats (centre) to form out-pouchings on the external (serosal) surface of the organ. These glands (Rokitansky-Aschoff sinuses) are probably still connected with the lumen and their epithelium is of normal adult form. **5.31 Primary carcinoma: gallbladder.** The tumour is a papilliferous columnar cell adenocarcinoma. The lumen is at the left, out of the picture, and only part of the thick carcinomatous epithelium that lined the organ can be seen here. The malignant glands are of very variable size and shape and are growing through the hypertrophied muscle coat to the subserosa (right). The largest of the glands shows clearly the papilliferous form of the neoplasm. Gallbladder carcinoma usually resembles bile duct carcinoma and in 90 per cent of cases gall-stones are present. From this it has been inferred that gall-stones predispose to the development of carcinoma. **5.32 Acute haemorrhagic pancreatitis.** The condition is thought to result from release and activation of pancreatic enzymes, particularly lipase and trypsin, but though it is occasionally associated with cholelithiasis, the exact pathogenesis is obscure. In this field there is a focus of fat necrosis. The

fatty tissue has completely disintegrated and only cell debris and haemorrhage remain. The blue colour (below) is caused by deposition of calcium salts which occurs very rapidly. The necrotising process is beginning to affect the exocrine tissue on the left. **5.33 Diffuse chronic sclerosing pancreatitis.** Fibrous tissue has formed around and within the pancreatic lobules. The fibrous tissue contains a mixture of lymphocytes, plasma cells and polymorphs. The exocrine glands are somewhat distorted and the size of the lumen is increased. The epithelial cells are cuboidal rather than columnar and presumably have lost some of their enzyme-secreting powers. They show no nuclear abnormality, however, and the lesion should not be mistaken for carcinoma. **5.34 Atrophy: pancreas.** A calculus blocked the main pancreatic duct. The exocrine tissue has been replaced by fat and loose connective tissue. The endocrine tissue is unaffected and the islets of Langerhans even appear to be increased in number, because of the shrinkage of the organ. In effect this is a 'Banting and Best pancreas'. **5.35 Mucoviscidosis (fibrocystic disease): pancreas.** The ductules and acini are distended with dense laminated secretion and lined by flat and atrophic cells. Fibrous tissue is greatly increased in and around the lobule. Pancreatic achylia is an important feature of this disease which affects many other systems. The basic fault may be in the synthesis of epithelial mucins, leading to an increase in the consistence of the epithelial secretions. Even if the infant survives the neonatal period the prognosis is poor. **5.36 Primary carcinoma: pancreas.** The tumour cells are very pleomorphic but form rudimentary acini, some of which resemble exocrine tissue. The stroma is abundant and densely fibrous. Carcinoma of pancreas is a common tumour, the majority arising in the head of the organ. Most seem to come from duct epithelium.

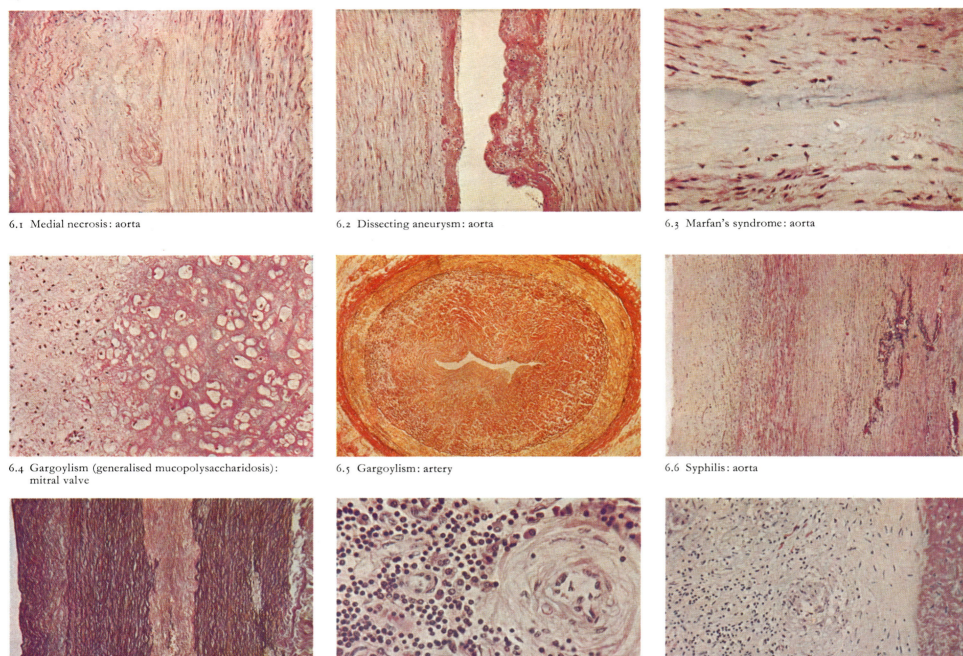

6.1 Medial necrosis: aorta

6.2 Dissecting aneurysm: aorta

6.3 Marfan's syndrome: aorta

6.4 Gargoylism (generalised mucopolysaccharidosis):
      mitral valve

6.5 Gargoylism: artery

6.6 Syphilis: aorta

6.7 Syphilis: aorta

6.8 Syphilis: aorta

6.9 Gumma: heart

6.1 Medial necrosis: aorta. This shows the medial coat. There has been considerable replacement of the elastic and muscular tissue by 'loose' poorly cellular connective tissue; the mucinous ground-substance filling the spaces in this tissue is unstained. Disrupted elastic laminae are visible (left). These changes weaken the vessel wall and a dissecting aneurysm may develop, particularly when the patient is hypertensive. **6.2 Dissecting aneurysm: aorta.** The medial coat has been split by haemorrhage which entered through a slit-like opening in the ascending part of the arch. Most of the extravasated blood has been lost but a layer of red-staining fibrin lines the false channel (centre). The media shows some loss of muscle and elastic tissue and 'replacement' fibrosis is fairly marked. **6.3 Marfan's syndrome: aorta.** This shows part of the media. There is a greatly increased content of bluish-staining mucinous material and a considerable reduction in the amount of musculo-elastic tissue, with its complete disappearance in the central area. The vessel wall is correspondingly weakened. The aorta therefore tends to dilate and a dissecting aneurysm not infrequently develops. **6.4 Gargoylism (generalised mucopolysaccharidosis): mitral valve.** This shows one of the valve cusps. The connective tissue cells are characteristically swollen, with vacuolated cytoplasm, and between them there is a considerable amount of mucopolysaccharide (coloured purplish-red here by the periodic acid-Schiff technique). In this disease deposition of mucopolysaccharide occurs in many tissues. **6.5 Gargoylism: artery.** This is a coronary artery from the same case as in 6.4, stained by the van Gieson

method. The muscular media (coloured yellow) is of normal thickness but the lumen is reduced to a slit by a relatively enormous collagenous thickening of the intima. **6.6–6.8 Syphilis: aorta. 6.6** The whole thickness of the aortic wall is visible, with the lumen on the left. The vasa vasorum in the adventitia and media (right) are congested and surrounded by a cuff of blue-staining inflammatory cells. The normal tissues in the vicinity of these vessels have been destroyed, and the considerable loss of musculo-elastic tissue from the adjacent media (centre) is evident when it is compared with the more deeply staining media in the inner third of the vessel. The pale-staining tissue on the left of the latter is a thick and fibrous intima. **6.7** This is the same field as 6.6 stained to show elastic tissue. There has been considerable loss of elastic tissue from the centre of the media and also around the vasa vasorum. Loss of elastic tissue greatly weakens the vessel wall and predisposes to aneurysm formation. When the first part of the aortic arch is affected, incompetence of the aortic valve generally results. **6.8** This shows the adventitia in detail. It is heavily infiltrated with lymphocytes and plasma cells, and the lumen of the small artery (right) has been greatly narrowed by endarteritis obliterans. The medial tissue supplied by this vessel would clearly tend to become ischaemic. **6.9 Gumma: heart.** The necrotic centre of the gumma is visible on the right. It is enclosed by granulation tissue which contains elongated histiocytes and many lymphocytes and plasma cells. The histiocytes resemble epithelioid cells and in one place they form a small follicle (centre).

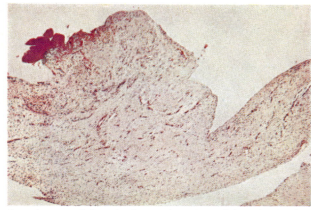

6.10 Acute and chronic rheumatic endocarditis: mitral valve

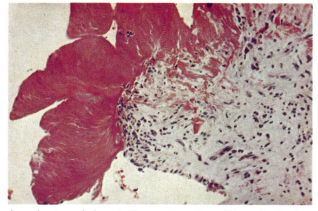

6.11 Acute and chronic rheumatic endocarditis: mitral valve

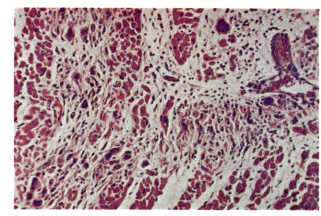

6.12 Acute rheumatic myocarditis

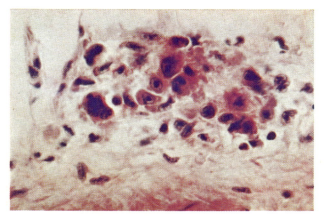

6.13 Acute rheumatic myocarditis

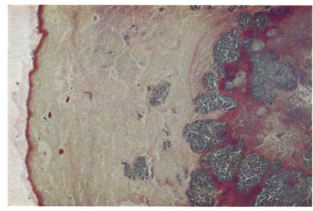

6.14 Subacute bacterial endocarditis: aortic valve

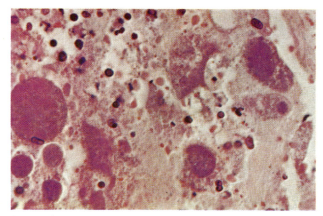

6.15 Q fever: aortic valve

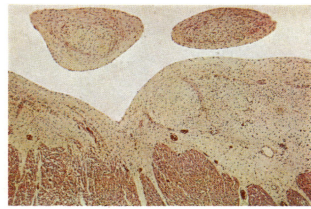

6.16 Congenital endocardial fibroelastosis of infants

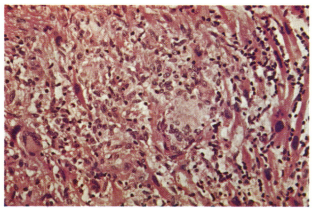

6.17 Giant cell myocarditis

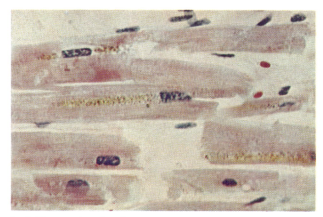

6.18 Brown atrophy: heart

6.10 and **6.11 Acute and chronic rheumatic endocarditis: mitral valve. 6.10** This is the distal half of a mitral valve cusp. The cusp is thick, fibrous and vascular as a result of previous attacks of acute rheumatic endocarditis (valvulitis). There is also evidence of an active rheumatic process in the form of a small red-stained vegetation near the tip of the cusp, on the line of closure (top left). **6.11** This shows the vegetation in more detail. It forms an eosinophilic mass which is believed to consist mainly of fused platelets. The vegetation, which is closely adherent to the thickened valve cusp, is being invaded and 'organised' by macrophages and fibroblasts. There are also a few lymphocytes and plasma cells. Complete organisation of the vegetation produces a fibrous scar and valvular stenosis and/or incompetence. **6.12** and **6.13 Acute rheumatic myocarditis. 6.12** There are several Aschoff nodules in the loose connective tissues of the myocardium, located characteristically near a small blood vessel (top right). The cells of each focus are mostly large and pleomorphic, and some are multinucleate. Their cytoplasm is basophilic. Between the cells there is eosinophilic material, generally considered to be necrotic connective tissue. The myocardial fibres are separated by inflammatory oedema and there is mild infiltration by small dark-staining cells. Some of the myocardial fibres appear degenerate, but though it has been suggested that the large cells in the Aschoff nodule are of myogenic origin this is unlikely. The Aschoff nodule, which is pathognomonic of acute rheumatic carditis, heals by fibrosis. **6.13** The mononuclear cells which make up this discrete Aschoff nodule resemble macrophages but they have larger nuclei and show considerable pleomorphism. The nucleoli are particularly prominent. **6.14 Subacute bacterial endocarditis: aortic valve.** This is part of one of the large vegetations that were present on an aortic cusp. There are large

numbers of degenerate polymorphs (left) and pink-staining material which is a mixture of platelets and fibrin (centre and right). Colonies of bacteria (in this instance, *Streptococcus viridans*) are present within this material (e.g. middle right and top right). Vegetations of this type are soft and readily give rise to emboli. **6.15 Q fever: aortic valve.** This is a section of one of the vegetations which was present on the cusps of the aortic valve at necropsy. The diagnostic feature is the presence of macrophages (left edge) greatly swollen from the presence within them of enormous numbers of very small bluish-staining organisms *(Coxiella burnetii)*. A few lymphocytes are also seen. The pale-staining material between the cells consists mainly of fused platelets. **6.16 Congenital endocardial fibroelastosis of infants.** In this low-power view the myocardium is visible at the bottom. On its endocardial surface there is a thick layer of pale-staining connective tissue. This gave the endocardium a smooth porcelain-like appearance at necropsy. At the top, two thickened and fibrosed trabeculae carneae are seen in cross-section. **6.17 Giant cell myocarditis.** The myocardial fibres are displaced and in places disrupted by the presence of mononuclear cells and multinucleated giant cells (right of centre and lower left corner). Before a diagnosis of giant cell myocarditis is made, known causes of granulomatous inflammation such as sarcoidosis, tuberculosis or syphilis should be excluded. **6.18 Brown atrophy: heart.** At necropsy the heart was small and lacked epicardial fat. There are collections of brown pigment (lipofuscin) in several myocardial fibres. These are located at the poles of the nuclei. The muscle fibres are narrower than normal. The fragmentation is artefactual. Brown atrophy generally occurs when death follows prolonged cachexia, as in malignant disease.

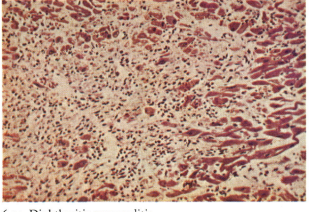

6.19 Diphtheritic myocarditis

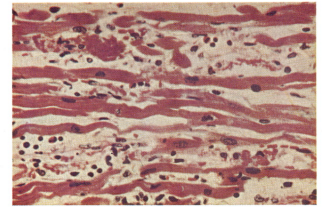

6.20 Diphtheritic myocarditis

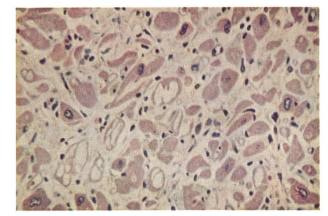

6.21 Mumps: myocarditis

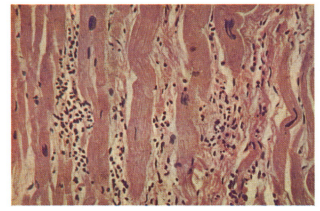

6.22 Isolated (viral?) myocarditis

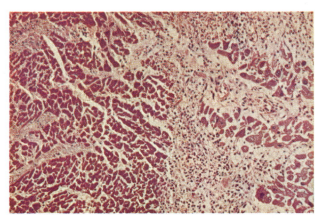

6.23 Infarct: heart

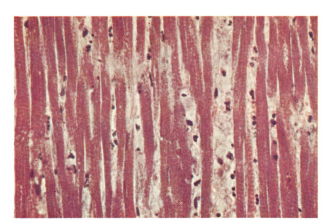

6.24 Infarct: heart

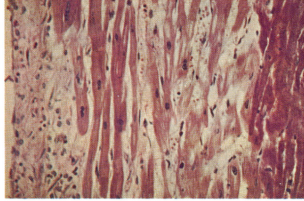

6.25 Infarct: heart

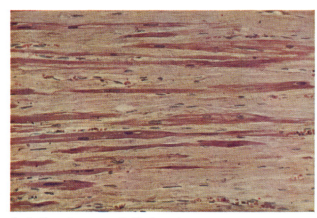

6.26 Chronic myocardial ischaemia

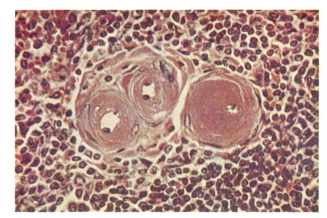

6.27 Arteriolosclerosis

6.19 and **6.20 Diphtheritic myocarditis. 6.19** There is considerable destruction of muscle cells and many chronic inflammatory cells are present in the interstitial tissues. Lesions of this sort were scattered throughout the heart but much of the myocardium showed no change. **6.20** The muscle fibres show varying degrees of damage, ranging from loss of striations up to complete necrosis and fragmentation. Interstitial oedema is evident. The cellular infiltrate is slight, most of the cells being lymphocytes though a few eosinophils are also present. **6.21** and **6.22 Viral myocarditis.** In 6.21 the mump virus was responsible; in 6.22 a viral etiology was assumed on clinical evidence. **6.21** The myocardial fibres stain very poorly and show degenerative and atrophic changes. Many contain large central vacuoles. Others, perhaps less affected, have abnormally large nuclei. The interstitial tissues are oedematous and contain necrotic cellular debris. In other parts of the heart, necrosis of fibres was a very marked feature. It is possible that the vacuolation of fibres was due to potassium toxicity. **6.22** Some of the muscle fibres are swollen and show loss of striations. Others show foci of necrosis and in these areas there is an infiltrate of inflammatory cells, both mononuclear and polymorph. **6.23–6.25 Infarct: heart. 6.23** This is the edge of an infarct one week old. The dead muscle (left) stains deeply and lacks nuclei. Between the living muscle (right) and the dead muscle there is a zone rich in polymorphs, macrophages and fibroblasts. When the patient with a lesion like this survives, the phagocytes digest the dead muscle and the fibroblasts form a fibrous scar. **6.24** This is the dead muscle. The fibres are still striated but deeply eosinophilic and without nuclei. Many of the cells in the interstitial tissue are also necrotic, but some have intact nuclei and are probably macrophages which have penetrated into the dead tissue. **6.25** This is the endocardial surface. The necrotic myocardial fibres (right) are deep-staining and lack nuclei but beneath the endocardium (left) a thin layer of muscle remains viable. The fibres here are nucleated but stain very palely. Considerable oedema is present in and around them. They have survived because of their close proximity to the blood in the ventricle. **6.26 Chronic myocardial ischaemia.** The patient had severe atherosclerosis and narrowing of the coronary arteries. Many muscle fibres have disappeared and been replaced by dense, poorly cellular fibrous tissue. Some of the surviving muscle fibres appear hypertrophied with very large basophilic nuclei but most are small and atrophic. **6.27 Arteriolosclerosis.** These are splenic arterioles. In the subendothelium of each there is a mass of acellular hyaline material which has narrowed the lumen to a considerable degree. The muscle cells in the media are intact but atrophic. The splenic cells are lymphocytes. This type of lesion is often seen in older subjects but it occurs earlier and more severely in hypertension. The other organs usually affected are kidney, pancreas and liver.

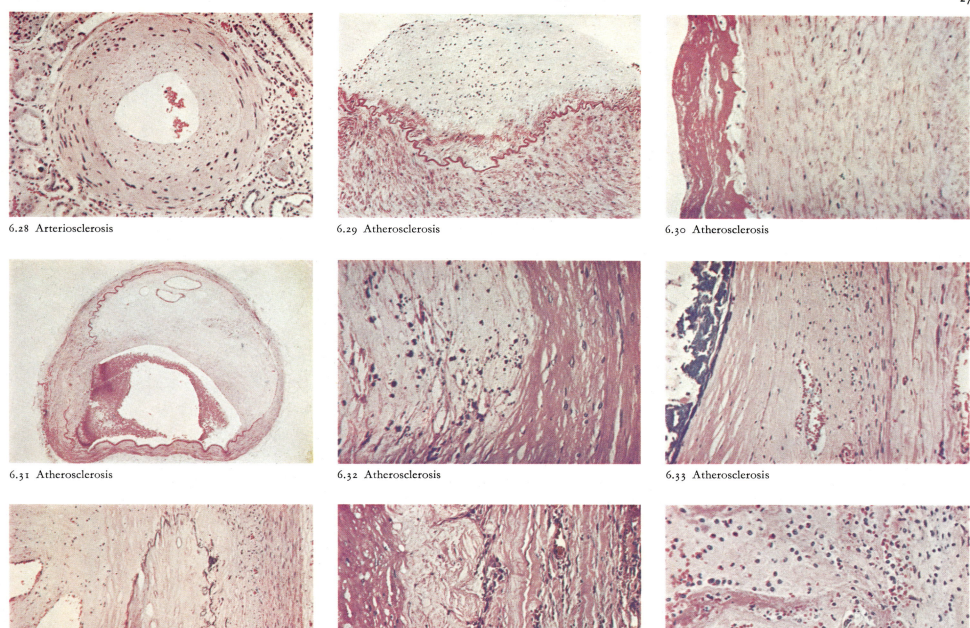

6.28 Arteriosclerosis

6.29 Atherosclerosis

6.30 Atherosclerosis

6.31 Atherosclerosis

6.32 Atherosclerosis

6.33 Atherosclerosis

6.34 Atherosclerosis

6.35 Aneurysm femoral artery

6.36 Thrombosis: coronary artery

6.28 Arteriosclerosis. The patient was both hypertensive and diabetic. In this arcuate artery in the kidney, many of the muscle cells in the hypertrophied media have been replaced by fibrous tissue. The intima is very thick and fibrous, with consequent reduction in the lumen. The internal elastic lamina has fragmented in many places. **6.29–6.34 Atherosclerosis. 6.29** This early lesion in the aorta is a small cushion-shaped plaque of avascular myxoid connective tissue (top). The small collection of large cells with clear cytoplasm deep in the plaque are lipid-laden phagocytes (left of centre). The underlying elastic lamina is depressed but intact. The media (bottom is slightly atrophied. **6.30** This shows the thickened fibrous intima (middle and right) of an atherosclerotic aorta. On the intimal surface there is a plaque of fibrin (left) which is beginning to acquire a covering of endothelium. The large cells lying between the fibrin and the intima are probably macrophages breaking down the fibrin. Organisation and incorporation of a fibrin plaque like this is one way in which the atherosclerotic intimal thickening may develop (fibrin encrustation theory). Many of the large cells in the intima are probably smooth muscle cells. **6.31** This is a coronary artery. Severe atherosclerosis has greatly reduced the lumen. The internal elastic lamina underlying the plaque has disappeared and the adjacent media is thin and atrophic 6.32 and 6.33 are taken from the deeper parts of a large plaque in the femoral artery. **6.32** Here the plaque consists of loose connective tissue (left) and dense fibrous tissue (right). The clefts in the loose tissue contained crystals of cholesterol and fatty acids which dissolved during processing and a frozen section revealed considerable amounts of lipid. Closely associated with each cleft is a layer of fibrin. On the right an intact internal elastic lamina and atrophic media are visible. **6.33** Here the plaque consists of dense fibrous tissue and a mass of calcified debris (left). The capillaries (centre) have entered the plaque from the fibrosed media (right). The internal elastic lamina has disappeared. It should be noted that the clefts in the dense fibrous tissue are not crystal clefts but gaps produced in the dense fibrous tissue by shrinkage during processing of the tissue. **6.34** This is a coronary artery that had thrombosed three months prior to death. Partial recanalisation has occurred and the thrombus which occluded the artery has been organised and replaced by connective tissue through which run large vascular channels (left). A few capillaries are running from the atrophic media (right) into the thick, fibrous and partly calcified atheromatous intima (centre and right). **6.35 Aneurysm: femoral artery.** The severely atherosclerotic and weakened vessel has expanded to form a fusiform aneurysm, the wall of which consists only of dense fibrous tissue (right). The aneurysm is lined by thrombus (left) which is full of lipid in its deeper parts (left of centre). Note the many cholesterol clefts in this lipid-rich zone. A few lymphocytes accompany the capillaries in the fibrous wall of the aneurysm. **6.36 Thrombosis: coronary artery.** The patient died 4 hours after the onset of the attack. Thrombus is adherent to the fibrous atherosclerotic intima (right). The thrombus contains fibrin but most of it consists of platelets which lie in granular masses that stain less intensely than fibrin. Red cells are present in relatively small numbers and many of the trapped leucocytes are eosinophils.

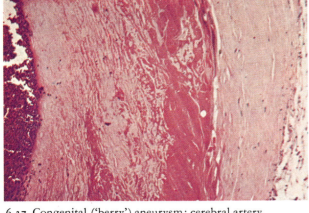

6.37 Congenital ('berry') aneurysm: cerebral artery

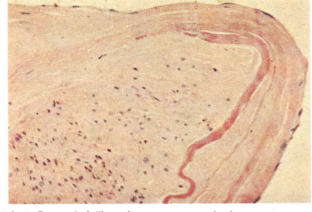

6.38 Congenital ('berry') aneurysm: cerebral artery

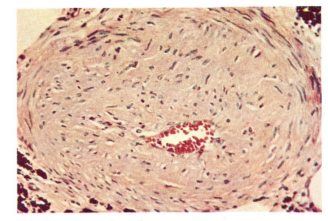

6.39 Mitral stenosis: pulmonary artery

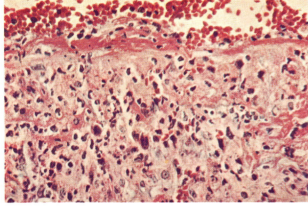

6.40 Mitral stenosis: pulmonary artery

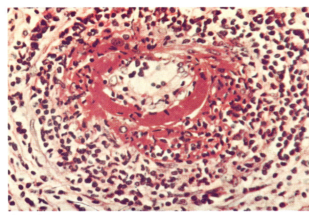

6.41 Acute arteritis

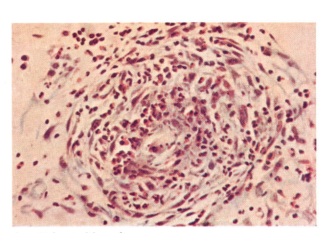

6.42 Polyarteritis nodosa

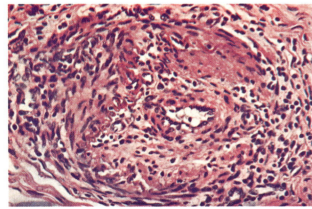

6.43 Polyarteritis nodosa

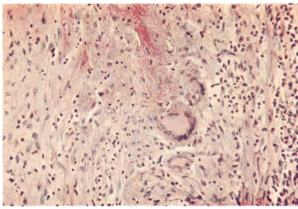

6.44 Temporal (giant-cell) arteritis

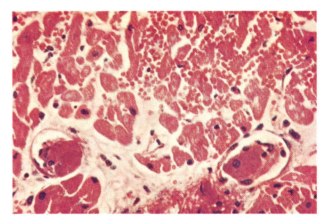

6.45 Thrombotic thrombocytopenic purpura (thrombotic micro-angiopathy)

6.37 and 6.38 Congenital ('berry') aneurysm: cerebral artery. 6.37 The wall consists of dense, hyaline fibrous tissue (right) and the lumen (left) contains a great deal of thrombus which appears to be mostly fibrin. There is extensive calcification (extreme left) within the thrombus. **6.38** This is the same aneurysm as 6.37. The lumen of the aneurysm is at the top and the stoma is at the top right corner. The media (below left) is fibrotic and the intima (right) is thick and fibrous. The swollen internal elastic lamina runs up to the stoma where it terminates. The wall of the aneurysm (top left) consists of hyaline fibrous tissue. Berry aneurysms are believed to arise on the basis of a defect in the muscular media, generally at bifurcations of the artery, but hypertension is often a predisposing factor. Rupture of the aneurysm leads to subarachnoid haemorrhage. **6.39 and 6.40 Mitral stenosis: pulmonary artery. 6.39** This small branch is hypertrophied as a result of pulmonary hypertension. The media and the intima are both greatly thickened and the lumen is correspondingly small. Many of the cells in the thickened intima appear to be smooth muscle cells. There are dust-filled macrophages in the adventitia. Severely affected vessels are generally atherosclerotic. **6.40** Rarely, as here, the muscle coat of the artery disintegrates, leaving a disordered mass of cells and necrotic fibrinoid material. Some of the cells are probably surviving smooth muscle cells but many are inflammatory and include macrophages, lymphocytes and polymorphs. There are some nuclear fragments. The endothelial cells have sloughed off and fibrin lines the vessel (top). **6.41 Acute arteritis.** This is a small muscular artery in the wall of the uterus and the lesion was an incidental finding. There is complete destruction of the arterial wall and replacement by inflammatory cells and red fibrinoid material within which there are nuclear fragments. The inflammatory cells are a mixture of macrophages, polymorphs and lymphocytes.

A few smooth muscle cells may survive. The intimal lining consists of swollen cells, probably of endothelial origin. **6.42 and 6.43 Polyarteritis nodosa. 6.42** This is a small necrotic artery. There is practically no lumen and eosinophil and neutrophil leucocytes infiltrate the necrotic media. They are also numerous in the adventitia. The elongated cells are probably fibroblasts and their presence, along with the many eosinophils, suggest that the lesion has entered a subacute or 'healing' phase. **6.43** Necrotic cell fragments and fibrinoid material have disappeared, and the lesion is now in the healing phase. Parts of the muscular coat and internal elastic lamina survive (above and left) but elsewhere (below right) both have disappeared. The intima is very thick and fibrous and the lumen is consequently very small and perhaps non-functional. Inflammatory cells are still numerous in the adventitia but they are mostly lymphocytes. **6.44 Temporal (giant-cell) arteritis.** This is a comparatively early lesion. A zone of fibrinoid necrosis (top centre) in the media is surrounded by macrophages and the multinucleated cells that typify this lesion. A few eosinophilic fragments of elastic tissue are present and lymphocytes are numerous, particularly in the adventitia (right). **6.45 Thrombotic thrombocytopenic purpura (thrombotic micro-angiopathy).** This is the myocardium. Slight haemorrhage has occurred into the oedematous interstitial tissues but the most notable feature is the presence of thrombi within the capillaries. Similar microthrombi were present in other organs but none of the larger vessels was affected. Histochemical tests suggest that much, if not all, of the thrombus material is fibrin, and not degenerate red cells or platelets as previously believed. Characteristically, the patient was a girl of 16 who suffered from fever, purpura, haemolytic anaemia and vague neurological signs.

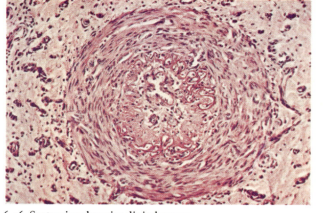

6.46 Systemic sclerosis: digital artery

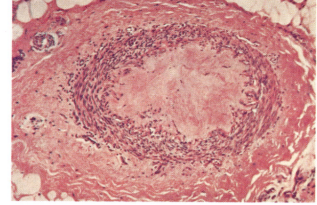

6.47 Systemic sclerosis: digital artery

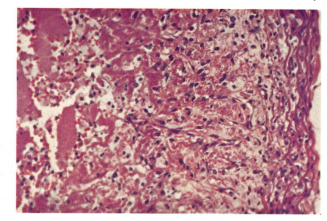

6.48 Organisation and recanalisation of thrombus

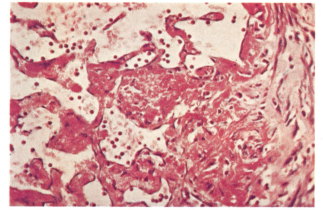

6.49 Organisation and recanalisation of thrombus

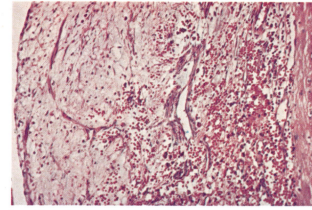

6.50 Organisation of mural thrombus

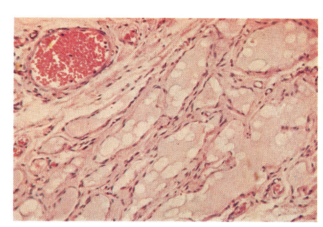

6.51 Cavernous lymphangioma

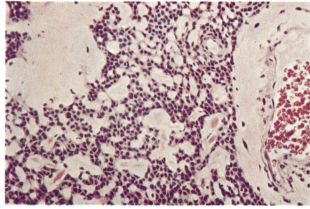

6.52 Glomangioma (glomus tumour)

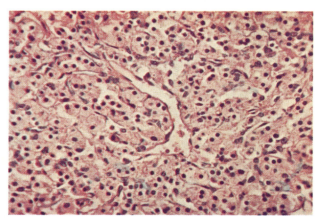

6.53 Carotid body tumour

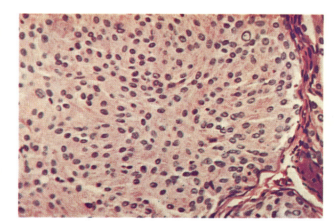

6.54 Glomus jugulare tumour

6.46 and **6.47 Systemic sclerosis: digital artery. 6.46** The artery is from a finger that became gangrenous at the tip. The media and the intima are both very thick and the lumen is very small. The greatly convoluted appearance of the internal elastic lamina, which is broken in two places, suggests that the artery has contracted to a marked extent. The adventitial tissues are very fibrous and the vasa vasorum unusually prominent. Similar changes are found in other viscera. **6.47** Like 6.46 this is a digital artery from a gangrenous finger. The adventitia is very thick and fibrous and the lumen is blocked by dense hyaline collagen. The media is relatively normal. **6.48** and **6.49 Organisation and recanalisation of thrombus. 6.48** The lumen (left) is full of thrombus which is being invaded and organised by capillaries and fibroblasts from the media, the elastic fibres of which are visible on the right. Foamy (lipid-laden) phagocytes (left) are present. **6.49** In this small vein organisation has proceeded much further. The capillaries which invaded the thrombus are now widely patent and have converted the thrombus into a spongy mass through which blood was probably able to flow slowly. The contents of the vascular channels are normal blood elements, including leucocytes and red cells. The wall of the vein is visible on the right. **6.50 Organisation of mural thrombus.** The patient had atrial fibrillation and this is part of the smooth glistening thrombus that was firmly adherent to the wall of the left auricle. Most of the thrombus has been organised with formation of a considerable amount of myxoid connective tissue (left) over which endothelium has grown. At least some 'myxomas' of heart are organised mural thrombi. **6.51 Cavernous lymphangioma.** The

lesion, which was in the skin, consists of thick-walled vascular channels lined by endothelium and filled with lymph. A small vein is visible (top left). Many lymphangiomas are congenital. **6.52 Glomangioma (glomus tumour).** The lesion, which was located characteristically in the nail-bed, consists of compact masses and cords of small polyhedral cells with relatively large nuclei of uniform size and shape. The abundant intercellular substance is almost colourless but often it stains well with eosin. The tumour bears some resemblance to a sweat gland adenoma but it is derived from the glomus cells which are located in the walls of small arteries in arteriovenous shunts and which are supposed by their contractile powers to regulate the blood-flow. The vessel on the right is a small artery. **6.53 Carotid body tumour.** This is a non-chromaffin paraganglioma or chemodectoma. The uniform large polygonal cells, which have abundant eosinophilic cytoplasm and dark-staining nuclei, enclose a very extensive network of vessels which have collapsed during removal and processing. A reticulin stain would show an alveolar pattern that is an aid to diagnosis. Though the tumour is benign, the location next to the bifurcation of the carotid artery makes resection difficult. **6.54 Glomus jugulare tumour.** This is another example of non-chromaffin paraganglioma or chemodectoma. The tumour cells form a spherical mass which is enclosed in vascular fibrous tissue (right). The tumour comes from the cells of the glomus body in the adventitia of the bulb of the jugular vein. It is histologically identical with the carotid body tumour but differs from it in being locally invasive and destructive.

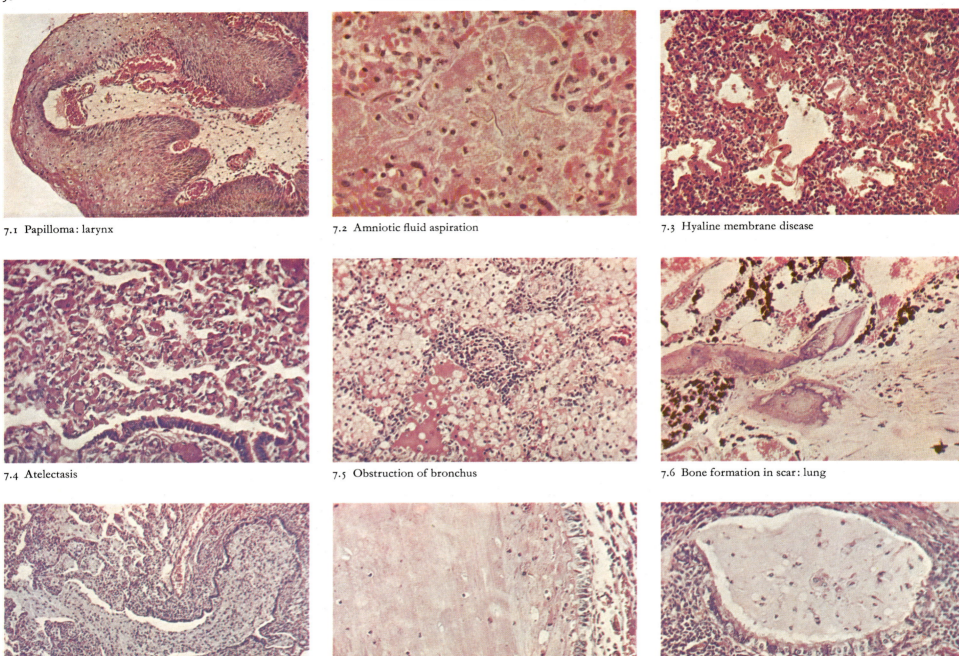

7.1 Papilloma: larynx

7.2 Amniotic fluid aspiration

7.3 Hyaline membrane disease

7.4 Atelectasis

7.5 Obstruction of bronchus

7.6 Bone formation in scar: lung

7.7 Mucoviscidosis: lung

7.8 Mucoviscidosis: lung

7.9 Mucoviscidosis: lung

7.1 Papilloma: larynx. The epithelium of the papilloma is thick and hyperplastic and shows a tendency to keratinisation. The deeper cells have large active-looking nuclei and occasional mitotic figures are present. The stroma of the tumour consists of oedematous and vascular areolar tissue infiltrated with scanty lymphocytes. In children these lesions tend to recur. They may also disappear spontaneously. A virus may be responsible. **7.2 Amniotic fluid aspiration.** This is the lung of a new-born child. The alveoli are full of granular coagulated protein and epithelial squames. There are also neutrophil leucocytes, suggestive of fetal pneumonia. The granular material and squames have come from inhaled amniotic fluid. The alveolar capillaries are congested. **7.3 Hyaline membrane disease.** The infant died 30 hours after delivery by Caesarean section. The pulmonary alveoli are collapsed and densely staining hyaline membrane lines the dilated alveolar ducts. The air present has tended to press the membrane against the alveolar wall. The lung is congested and there is perivascular oedema. **7.4 Atelectasis.** This is the lung of an infant who lived for only a few hours. The alveoli (top) supplied by the bronchiole (bottom) have failed to expand. The capillaries are engorged. **7.5 Obstruction of bronchus.** This shows consolidated lung distal to a carcinoma which was blocking a segmental bronchus. The alveoli are full of foamy (lipid-laden) macrophages and a deeply-staining (probably protein-rich) fluid. There are also considerable numbers of dark-staining plasma cells and lymphocytes. The

lipid in the macrophages gave the lesion a yellow colour macroscopically, and this is sometimes accepted as endogenous lipid pneumonia, in contrast to the exogenous forms which are caused by inhalation of lipoid material. **7.6 Bone formation in lung scar.** Bone trabeculae have formed within a small dense fibrous scar. Dust-laden phagocytes are present in large numbers in the scar and in the surrounding tissues. The scar was located at the apex of the lung but the aetiology was not known. **7.7–7.9 Mucoviscidosis: lung.** In this disease a general abnormality of mucous secretion affects many systems. Sweat secretion is also abnormal. 7.7 Dense mucus fills a bronchiole and its associated alveoli. Many inflammatory cells are present in the mucus. 7.8 The mucosa of this small bronchus survives but is reduced to a single layer of cells. The lumen is full of eosinophilic secretion in which a small number of macrophages float. The mucoid secretion looks much denser than normal and rather like cartilage matrix. 7.9 Degeneration of the respiratory epithelium is even more advanced in this bronchiole which in one part (top) is reduced to an incomplete layer of flattened cells. The wall of the bronchiole is inflamed and fibrosed and heavily infiltrated with chronic inflammatory cells, mostly plasma cells. The lumen is full of basophilic mucus in which macrophages are suspended. One of these (below centre) is in mitosis. In mucoviscidosis purulent bronchitis and bronchiectasis generally supervene, and often the affected child dies of bronchopneumonia.

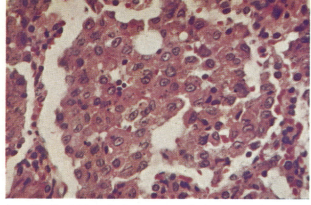

7.10 Kaolin (china-clay) pneumoconiosis

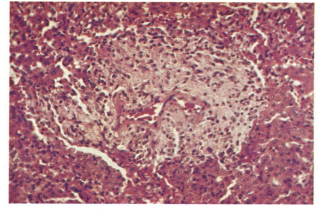

7.11 Kaolin pneumoconiosis

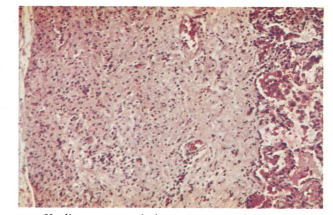

7.12 Kaolin pneumoconiosis

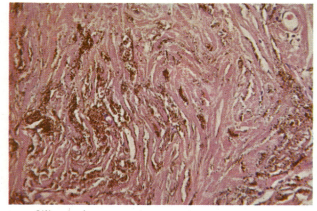

7.13 Silicosis: lung

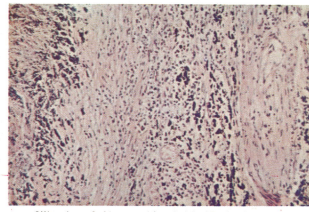

7.14 Silicosis and rheumatoid arthritis (Caplan lesion)

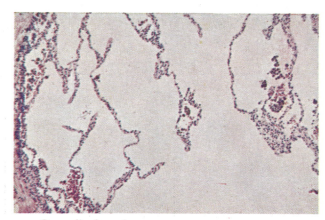

7.15 Generalised emphysema

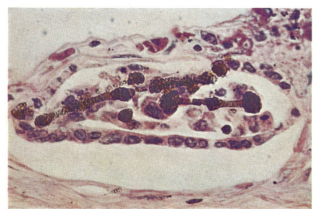

7.16 Asbestosis: lung

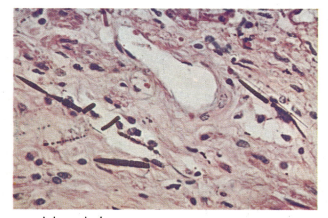

7.17 Asbestosis: lung

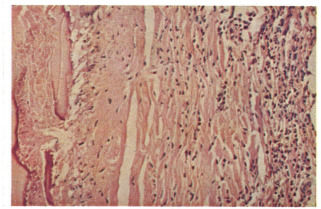

7.18 Hydatid disease (echinococcosis): lung

7.10–7.12 Kaolin (china-clay) pneumoconiosis. 7.10 This is one of many alveoli full of large dust-laden macrophages. The dust does not appear to be toxic and the macrophages show no signs of degeneration; nor is there evidence of fibrosis. The walls of the alveoli are slightly compressed. **7.11** Though the dust does not appear to be toxic for macrophages, this small vessel has a cuff of cellular fibrous tissue in which a considerable amount of dust is present. The surrounding alveoli contain large numbers of dust-filled cells. **7.12** There is considerable fibrous thickening of the visceral pleura. The cellular fibrous tissue contains a great deal of kaolin dust and the underlying alveoli (right) are full of dust-laden phagocytes. **7.13 Silicosis: lung.** This is part of one of the many hard nodules that were scattered throughout both lungs. It consists of extremely dense, virtually acellular, hyalinised fibrous tissue. Very few blood vessels are present. The brown pigment is coal-dust, the highly fibrogenic silica dust being colourless and invisible. The cracks in the fibrous tissue are caused by shrinkage during processing. **7.14 Silicosis and rheumatoid arthritis (Caplan lesion).** This is the edge of a pulmonary silicotic nodule. The nodule is necrotic (left) and surrounded by an infiltrate of plasma cells, lymphocytes, fibroblasts and dust-laden macrophages (centre). The blood vessel (right) is sclerotic and narrowed and its intimal coat contains plasma cells and lymphocytes. **7.15 Generalised emphysema.** The pleura is on the left. The alveolar walls are thin and atrophic and in places have broken down to form bullae. There are a few small collections of pigment-laden macrophages in the alveoli. In generalised emphysema the alveolar ducts and sacs are uniformly enlarged throughout the lungs and there

is no great variation from lobule to lobule. In centrilobular emphysema, however, the spaces are larger and the lesions are irregular in distribution and intensity. To diagnose emphysema it is best to fix the lungs in an expanded position so that the interlobular septa can be identified and their relationship to the emphysematous spaces established by whole lung sections and low-power microscopy. **7.16** and **7.17 Asbestosis: lung.** Several 'asbestos bodies' are present within a terminal bronchiole. These are asbestos fibrils (crystals of magnesium silicate) which are coated with protein- and iron-containing material. Macrophages are present round the bodies and dense fibrous tissue has formed round the bronchiole. The gap between epithelium and fibrous tissue has been produced by shrinkage during processing. **7.17** Asbestos fibrils are enclosed in dense fibrous tissue. Some have been dislodged during section cutting, leaving empty lacunae. One fibril is uncoated and shows the normal clear refractile structure of an asbestos crystal. The pleura is usually severely affected in asbestosis and the disease predisposes to the development not only of bronchial carcinoma but also of pleural mesothelioma. **7.18 Hydatid disease (echinococcosis): lung.** This is the outer part of the cyst wall. On the left is the cuticular layer which consists of amorphous, densely laminated chitinous material which is being digested by macrophages. This is enclosed by the adventitious layer, consisting of fibrous tissue in which there are many eosinophils. The inner germinative layer is not shown here. The cysts may be found in lung, liver, brain or bone, and form slowly-growing space-occupying lesions. The adult worm is a very small Cestode, 3–5 mm. long, consisting of only a few segments and its normal host is the dog.

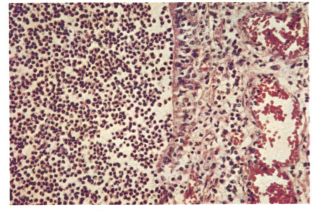

7.19 Acute bronchitis

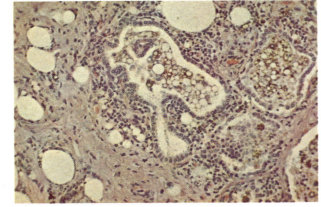

7.20 Lipid (aspiration) pneumonia

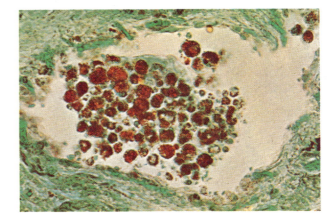

7.21 Lipid (aspiration) pneumonia

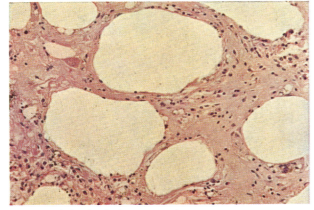

7.22 Lipid (aspiration) pneumonia

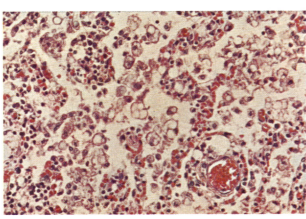

7.23 Lipid (aspiration) pneumonia

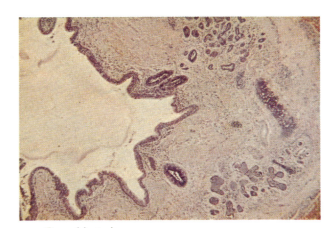

7.24 Bronchiectasis

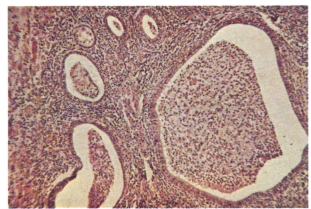

7.25 Bronchiectasis

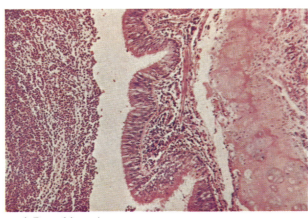

7.26 Bronchiectasis

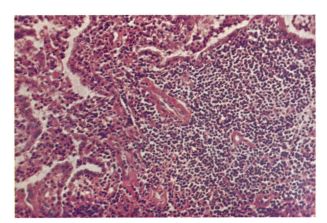

7.27 Bronchiectasis

7.19 Acute bronchitis. The mucosa is acutely inflamed and polymorphs are migrating through the respiratory epithelium (centre) from the dilated vessels in the mucosa into the lumen (left) which is full of pus. Fibrin strands are visible beneath the epithelium, in the lamina propria. **7.20–7.23 Lipid (aspiration) pneumonia. 7.20** The lesions are from the lungs of a patient who for many years used nose drops with a mineral oil base. The bronchioles are filled with foamy (lipoid) material and the adjacent alveoli have been replaced by inflammatory cells and fibrous tissue in which large lipoid droplets have been trapped. This lesion is sometimes called a 'paraffinoma'. **7.21** This is a frozen section which has been stained with Sudan IV to demonstrate the lipoid contents of the macrophages in the lumen of a small bronchus. **7.22** The lung parenchyma has been replaced by dense fibrous tissue. The large spaces contained mineral oil which has been lost during processing. **7.23** This is a less severely affected part of the lung. Within the pulmonary alveoli there are large numbers of macrophages with vacuolated cytoplasm. The vacuoles contained mineral oil. The lung is congested and there is evidence of more acute inflammatory

reaction in the form of clusters of small darkly-stained polymorphs. **7.24–7.27 Bronchiectasis. 7.24** The bronchus is greatly dilated but it is still lined by respiratory epithelium. However, the mucosa (right) is fibrosed and infiltrated with chronic inflammatory cells. There has also been considerable destruction of cartilage and only small plaques (middle right) remain between the mucous glands. The muscle fibres are hypertrophied. The lumen contained muco-pus which was lost during processing. **7.25** The pleura is on the left. In place of the alveoli there is a chronic inflammatory exudate. The bronchioles are ectatic, pus-filled, and lined by non-ciliated columnar epithelium. **7.26** The dilated bronchus is full of pus but the ciliated respiratory epithelium (centre) survives and is even thicker than normal. The underlying lamina propria is infiltrated with inflammatory cells, most of which are plasma cells and lymphocytes. The cartilage (right) is undergoing absorption. **7.27** Inflammatory cells fill the terminal bronchioles (left), and in the adjacent tissues there are large collections of lymphocytes (right).

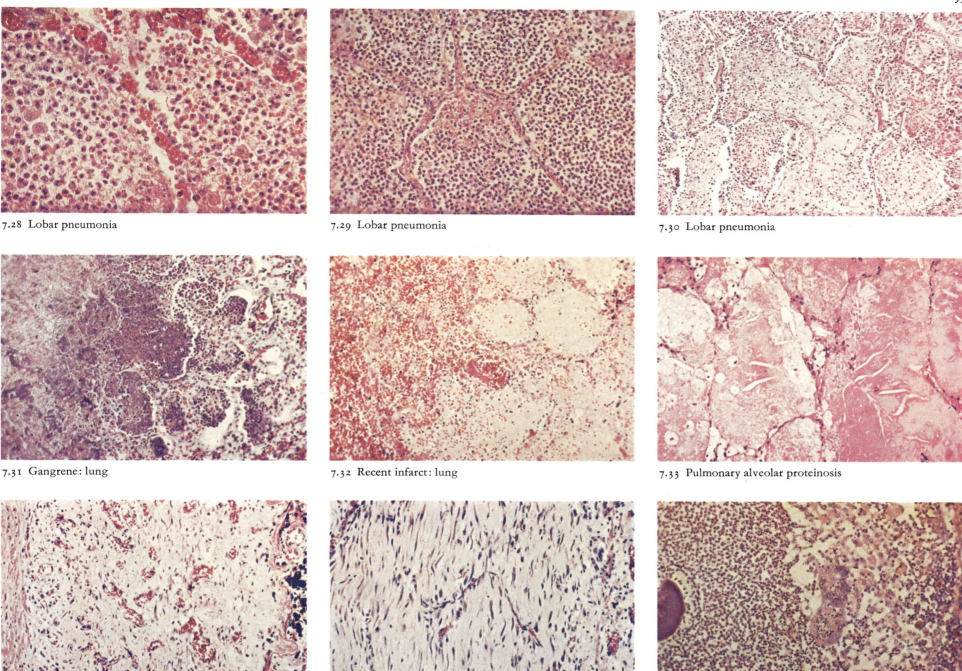

7.28 Lobar pneumonia

7.29 Lobar pneumonia

7.30 Lobar pneumonia

7.31 Gangrene: lung

7.32 Recent infarct: lung

7.33 Pulmonary alveolar proteinosis

7.34 Fibrinous pleurisy

7.35 Chronic fibrinous pleurisy

7.36 Actinomycotic abscess: lung

7.28–7.30 Lobar pneumonia. 7.28 The alveoli are filled with inflammatory exudate which consists largely of polymorphs though there are also red cells, degenerate macrophages and a little fibrin. The capillaries are still patent and macroscopically the lung showed red hepatisation. A Gram stain would probably demonstrate many pneumococci. **7.29** This is a later stage than 7.28. The exudate filling the alveoli is similar, consisting of polymorphs, fibrin and red cells, but the alveolar capillaries are much narrower. They are not completely collapsed, however, and the stage of grey hepatisation has not yet developed fully. **7.30** This is a still later stage of the pneumonic process and macroscopically the lung showed grey hepatisation. The exudate contains fewer polymorphs but more fibrin. However, the striking feature is the lack of blood in the alveolar capillaries. **7.31 Gangrene: lung.** Gangrene is generally taken to mean a combination of necrosis and putrefaction. Enormous numbers of micro-organisms (stained blue) are growing (left) in the lung which is necrotic and disintegrating. The concentration is very high in the advancing edge (centre) of the necrotising process. The adjacent lung (right) is acutely inflamed but still viable. **7.32 Recent infarct: lung.** The lung tissue (right) is necrotic and only nuclear fragments remain. There is extensive haemorrhage (left) and oedema (right). The patient had severe mitral stenosis and congestive heart failure. **7.33 Pulmonary alveolar proteinosis.** The

alveoli are full of dense pink exudate in which there are a few swollen macrophages. The clefts in the exudate contained cholesterol crystals which dissolved out during processing of the tissues. The alveolar walls and their capillaries are severely compressed. The aetiology of this condition is unknown. **7.34 Fibrinous pleurisy.** Only a little of the fibrinous exudate that covered the pleura remains (left), most of it having been organised and replaced by vascular granulation tissue. The serosal cells, which rested upon the layer of elastic tissue (right), have disappeared. **7.35 Chronic fibrinous pleurisy.** This is a later stage than 7.34. Organisation of the fibrinous exudate is complete and a layer of fibrous tissue has formed. This tissue is still cellular and fairly vascular. The elastic tissue of the pleura is visible (right). **7.36 Actinomycotic abscess: lung.** A mass of polymorphs surrounds the colony (left) of *Actinomyces israeli*. This collection of pus is bounded by vacuolated (lipid-laden) macrophages and lymphocytes (right), and a multinucleated giant macrophage which has nuclear debris in its cytoplasm is present. There are also a few haemosiderin-laden macrophages (right). The lipid-laden macrophages colour the pus particles yellow ('sulphur granules').

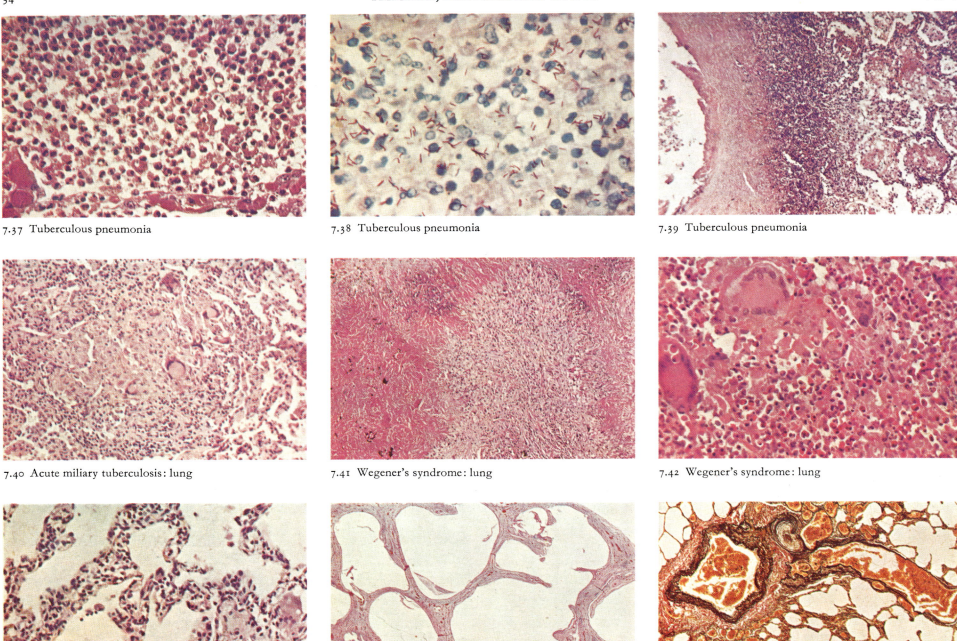

7.37 Tuberculous pneumonia

7.38 Tuberculous pneumonia

7.39 Tuberculous pneumonia

7.40 Acute miliary tuberculosis: lung

7.41 Wegener's syndrome: lung

7.42 Wegener's syndrome: lung

7.43 Extrinsic allergic alveolitis: lung

7.44 Systemic sclerosis: lung

7.45 Pulmonary hypertension: lung

7.37–7.39 Tuberculous pneumonia. 7.37 A vigorous inflammatory response has occurred and an inflammatory exudate which consists of macrophages and a lesser number of polymorphs fills the alveoli. Many of the macrophages are beginning to disintegrate. The alveolar capillaries (bottom) are acutely congested. **7.38** This is the same lesion as 7.37. A modified Ziehl-Neelsen stain reveals large numbers of acid-fast tubercle bacilli in the cytoplasm of the macrophages filling the alveoli. **7.39** The lung is consolidated. On the right the alveoli are filled with abundant pink-staining exudate containing small numbers of macrophages. On the left the consolidated lung has become necrotic (caseation); the caseous material has fragmented and been coughed up to leave a cavity. At the edge of the caseous area there is much blue-staining nuclear debris (centre). **7.40 Acute miliary tuberculosis: lung.** A miliary tubercle is present (centre). It consists of epithelioid cells and Langhans giant cells with numerous lymphocytes at the periphery. The adjacent alveoli are collapsed. Miliary tubercles generally start in the alveolar walls, where the bacterial emboli are filtered out of the blood stream. **7.41** and **7.42 Wegener's syndrome: lung. 7.41** The most prominent feature in this part of the lesion is the extensive necrosis. All the deeply eosinophilic tissue is necrotic, the only viable tissue being a cellular granulomatous tissue (centre and right of centre). Occasional giant cells can just be distinguished at the periphery of this granulomatous tissue. **7.42** This is a higher-power view of the granulomatous tissue in 7.41, showing several large multinucleated giant cells of Langhans type and large numbers of eosinophil polymorphs. **7.43 Extrinsic allergic alveolitis: lung.** The septa

are infiltrated with chronic inflammatory cells (lymphocytes, plasma cells and macrophages). There are also several multinucleated giant cells (right, centre) which formed part of a small follicle of the 'tuberculoid' type. In this instance the lung lesions resulted from reaction to a budgerigar's excretions, but similar changes can be produced by a variety of extrinsic allergens. Untreated allergic alveolitis generally leads to interstitial pulmonary fibrosis ('honeycomb' lung). **7.44 Systemic sclerosis: lung.** This is a very low-power view of the 'honeycomb' lung that sometimes develops in this disease, the result of interstitial pulmonary fibrosis. The normal lung architecture has been replaced by a series of relatively large air-filled spaces (several millimetres in diameter), the walls of which consist of vascular fibrous tissue. Closer examination would reveal the presence of numerous plasma cells and lymphocytes within the fibrous tissue and a cuboidal epithelium of 'bronchiolar' type lining the spaces. 'Honeycomb' lung has many causes but the changes are generally similar to those shown here. **7.45 Pulmonary hypertension: lung.** This section has been stained by an elastic-van Gieson method, which colours elastic tissue black and blood yellow. The patient suffered from patent ductus arteriosus and the changes present are the result of severe pulmonary hypertension. The pulmonary artery (upper left) shows marked medial thickening. Below and to the right of it are numerous abnormal vessels formed by dilatation of small branches of this artery. These thin-walled vessels form the so-called angiomatoid lesion. The prominent thin-walled vessel with the large lumen running to the right resembles a vein but is in fact a grossly dilated arteriole.

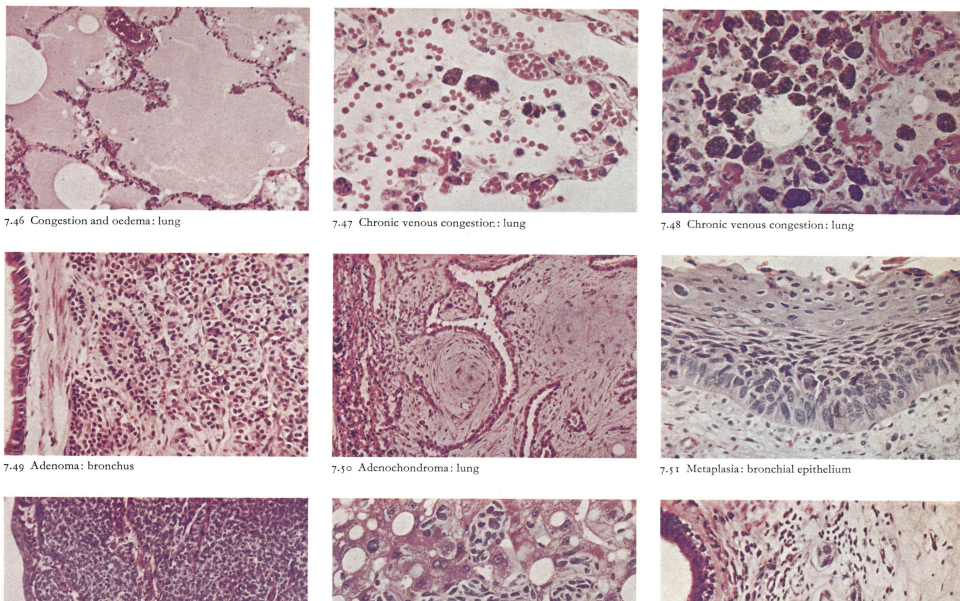

7.46 Congestion and oedema: lung

7.47 Chronic venous congestion: lung

7.48 Chronic venous congestion: lung

7.49 Adenoma: bronchus

7.50 Adenochondroma: lung

7.51 Metaplasia: bronchial epithelium

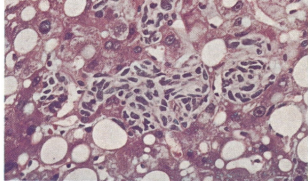

7.52 Primary undifferentiated ('oat-cell') carcinoma: bronchus

7.53 Secondary deposit of 'oat-cell' carcinoma: liver

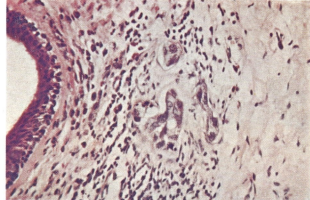

7.54 Spread of carcinoma by lymphatics: lung

7.46 Congestion and oedema: lung. The patient died of acute left ventricular failure. The alveolar capillaries are congested and the alveoli are filled with protein-rich fluid which is almost completely cell-free. The spaces are air trapped in the fluid. **7.47** and **7.48 Chronic venous congestion: lung.** In **7.47** the pulmonary capillaries are distended and tortuous and red cells have escaped from the vessels into the lumen of the alveolus where they mingle with macrophages. Several of the macrophages are very large and full of haemosiderin derived from red cells they have ingested. **7.48** This is a more severe and chronic lesion than **7.47**, the patient having had mitral stenosis for many years. The pulmonary capillaries are congested and varicose and within the alveoli are many macrophages so heavily laden with brown haemosiderin that their nuclei cannot be seen ('heart failure cells'). There is increase in fibrous tissue in the walls of the alveoli and this, combined with the abundant haemosiderin, is why the term 'brown induration' is applied to this lesion. **7.49 Adenoma: bronchus.** The ciliated respiratory epithelium is on the left. Beneath it, in the lamina propria, is a tumour mass consisting of solid masses and cords of epithelial cells. These cells have abundant cytoplasm and their nuclei are uniform in size and shape. Fibrous stroma is fairly scanty. The tumour cells are reminiscent of an argentaffinoma and occasionally an adenoma of bronchus is associated with the carcinoid syndrome. **7.50 Adenochondroma: lung.** Here the lesion consists of nodules of fibromyxomatous tissue and clefts

lined by bronchial epithelium. Elsewhere cartilage was present ('adeno-chondro-myxoma'). Lesions like this may enlarge but they are probably developmental anomalies. A few dust-laden cells are present in the pleura (left). **7.51 Metaplasia: bronchial epithelium.** The normal ciliated respiratory epithelium has been replaced by thick stratified squamous epithelium. This shows intense hyperplasia of the basal cells which are pleomorphic and possess large, hyperchromatic nuclei. Mitotic activity is considerable (left, for example). This type of lesion is common in cigarette smokers. **7.52 Primary undifferentiated ('oat-cell') carcinoma: bronchus.** The respiratory epithelium (left) is stretched over a mass of undifferentiated tumour consisting of uniform cells which have moderately sized nuclei and little cytoplasm. Mitotic figures are very numerous. The cells are close-packed and polyhedral in this primary mass. **7.53 Secondary deposit of 'oat-cell' carcinoma: liver.** The tumour has spread by the systemic circulation. The elongated shape of the tumour nuclei is obvious. Some of the liver cells show marked fatty change with the nucleus pushed to the periphery of the cell. **7.54 Spread of carcinoma by lymphatics.** This is the bronchial mucosa proximal to an undifferentiated primary carcinoma and malignant cells with large, pleomorphic nuclei are present in several mucosal lymphatics (centre). There is a lymphocytic and plasma cell response in the surrounding tissues and the basement membrane of the ciliated respiratory epithelium (left) is thicker than normal.

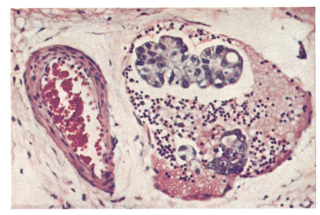

7.55 Spread of carcinoma by lymphatics: lung

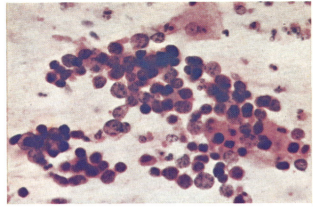

7.56 Primary carcinoma of bronchus: malignant cells in sputum

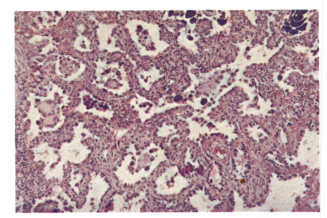

7.57 Alveolar carcinoma (pulmonary adenomatosis: bronchiolar carcinoma)

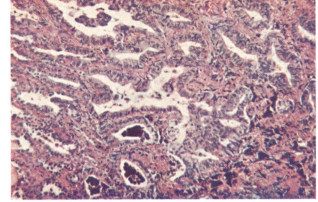

7.58 Alveolar carcinoma

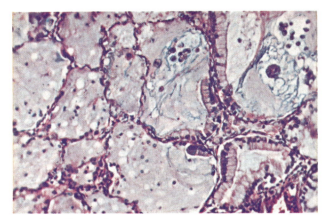

7.59 Alveolar carcinoma

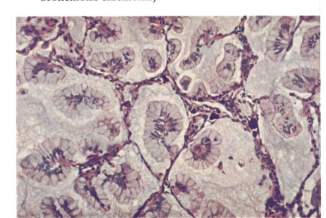

7.60 Alveolar carcinoma

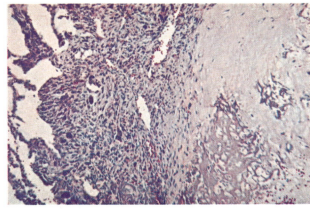

7.61 Secondary osteogenic sarcoma: lung

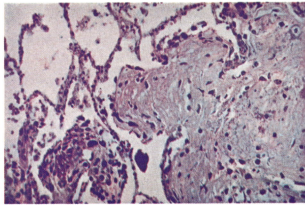

7.62 Secondary osteogenic sarcoma: lung

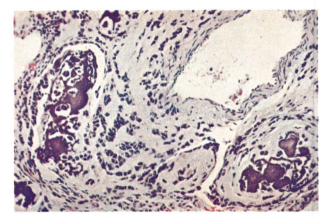

7.63 Secondary osteogenic sarcoma: lung

7.55 Spread of carcinoma by lymphatics: lung. The primary was an undifferentiated carcinoma of bronchus. Clumps of tumour cells float in the lymph in a peribronchial lymphatic channel (right). The lymph contains many lymphocytes. The other vessel (left) is a branch of the pulmonary artery. **7.56 Primary carcinoma of bronchus: malignant cells in sputum.** This is a smear of sputum. It shows clumps of undifferentiated cells which possess little or no cytoplasm. The large cells are squamous epithelial cells and a few polymorphs are also present. **7.57–7.60 Alveolar carcinoma (pulmonary adenomatosis; bronchiolar carcinoma).** This lesion is situated in a peripheral part of the lung, and no focus of origin in a bronchus can be demonstrated. It probably arises from the epithelium of the terminal bronchiole. The diagnosis is never certain without an autopsy to exclude the presence of a primary growth elsewhere. **7.57** The tumour cells are cuboidal and resemble bronchiolar epithelium and line spaces resembling alveoli. The appearance is like that produced by overgrowth of bronchiolar epithelium in and around a collapsed, fibrosed part of lung. Mucin secretion is not a feature of this particular neoplasm. Dust-laden macrophages as well as clumps of tumour cells are present within the 'alveoli'. **7.58** This is another part of the tumour shown in 7.57. Here the cells are much more obviously malignant being large columnar cells with pleomorphic and basophilic nuclei. They form irregular gland-like spaces which are in fact pulmonary alveoli, the cells having used the alveolar walls as their 'stroma'. The alveolar walls have also thickened and fibrosed. Some of these spaces contain clumps of dust-laden macrophages (bottom). There is a dust-laden scar (bottom right). **7.59** The tumour cells lining the pulmonary alveoli are tall goblet cells secreting great quantities of basophilic mucin that fills and distends the alveoli. A few macrophages float in the mucin. **7.60** This specimen also is secreting a great deal of mucin. The tumour cells are tall goblet cells which show a tendency to a papilliferous arrangement. A few dust-laden macrophages are present in the alveolar septa. **7.61–7.63 Secondary osteosarcoma: lung.** 7.61 shows the growing edge of a large deposit. The most superficial part (left) is intensely cellular, the malignant osteoblasts being large and very pleomorphic. Deeper in the deposit the cells have formed masses of pink uncalcified osteoid (top right) and blue calcified bone (bottom right). **7.62** In this part of the metastasis the neoplastic osteoblasts have formed only pink osteoid. **7.63** The vessel (top right) is a branch of the pulmonary artery and it is surrounded by secondary tumour. The neoplastic cells and their cytoplasm are typically basophilic. In several places (left and bottom right, for example) they have formed calcified bone matrix. The primary tumour, in a boy of 12, was at the lower end of femur.

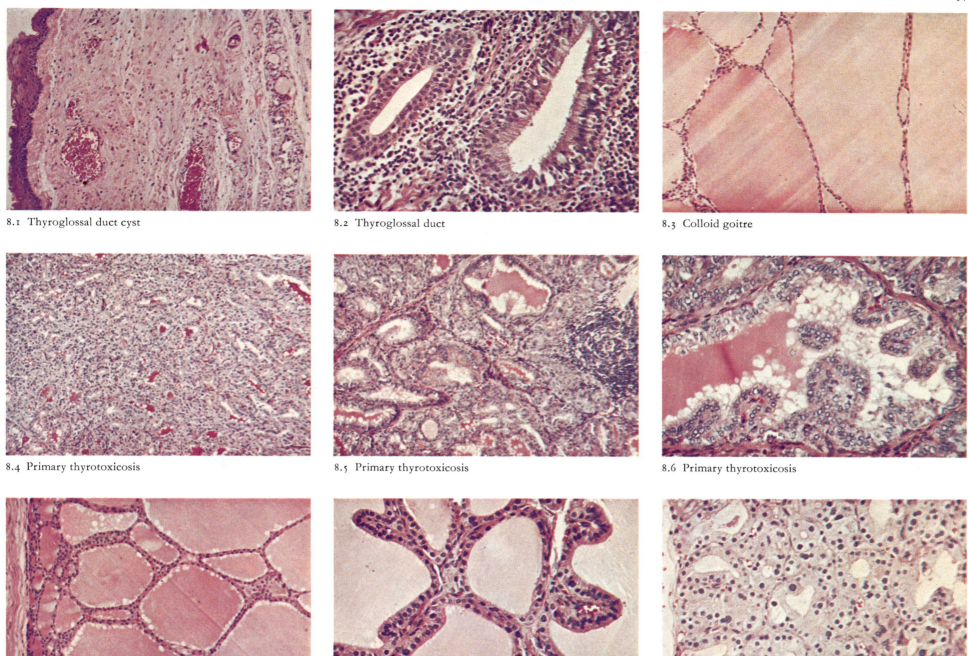

8.1 Thyroglossal duct cyst   8.2 Thyroglossal duct   8.3 Colloid goitre

8.4 Primary thyrotoxicosis   8.5 Primary thyrotoxicosis   8.6 Primary thyrotoxicosis

8.7 Primary thyrotoxicosis   8.8 Primary thyrotoxicosis   8.9 Primary thyrotoxicosis

8.1 and **8.2 Thyroglossal duct cyst. 8.1** This part of the cyst is lined with stratified squamous epithelium (left). The fibrous wall is vascular and contains some rather atrophic thyroid tissue (right). **8.2** At this point the duct is double. In one part (right) the epithelium is pseudostratified whereas in the other (left) it shows a tendency to a squamous form. Surrounding the ducts are plasma cells, lymphocytes and fibrous tissue. Branchial cleft cysts have a similar structure. **8.3 Colloid goitre.** The follicles are large or very large, full of colloid and lined by flattened epithelial cells. **8.4–8.9 Primary thyrotoxicosis.** In this form of hyperthyroidism the thyroid gland is diffusely enlarged. **8.4** The gland is intensely hyperplastic and cellular, consisting of small, closely-packed follicles. These are lined by columnar cells and colloid is very scanty within them. **8.5** Here the follicles vary considerably in size but generally tend to be small. The epithelium forms papilliform ingrowths into the larger follicles. There is some pale-staining colloid, perhaps as a result of pre-operative treatment with iodine. The colloid is vacuolated at the edges, a sign of active resorption. There is some increase of lymphoid tissue in the stroma (right). This is often a much more prominent feature. **8.6** This is a higher power view of the gland in 8.5 to show the tall, hyperplastic columnar epithelial cells and their marked tendency

to form papilliferous projections into the follicles. The colloid is pale-staining, scanty and excessively scalloped at the edges. The fibrous stroma is vascular, though increased vascularity is not always readily detected in histological sections since the small vessels tend to empty. **8.7** Pre-operative treatment with iodine has produced almost complete involution in this gland. The follicles are large, full of deeply-staining colloid, and lined by flattened epithelial cells. There is still some peripheral vacuolation of the colloid, showing that resorption of colloid continues. **8.8** This gland also shows involutionary change as a result of pre-operative treatment. The cells are now cuboidal and though a papilliform tendency is still present, the vesicles are large and well-filled with colloid. The colloid stains fairly well and vacuolation is absent. The gland is still hyperaemic. **8.9** This patient had been treated for some time with thiouracil, which tends to increase the degree of epithelial hyperplasia and decrease the storage of colloid. These features are evident here. Colloid is virtually absent and the follicles are lined by columnar cells the nuclei of which show considerable pleomorphism. This pleomorphism may suggest malignancy but there are no mitotic figures.

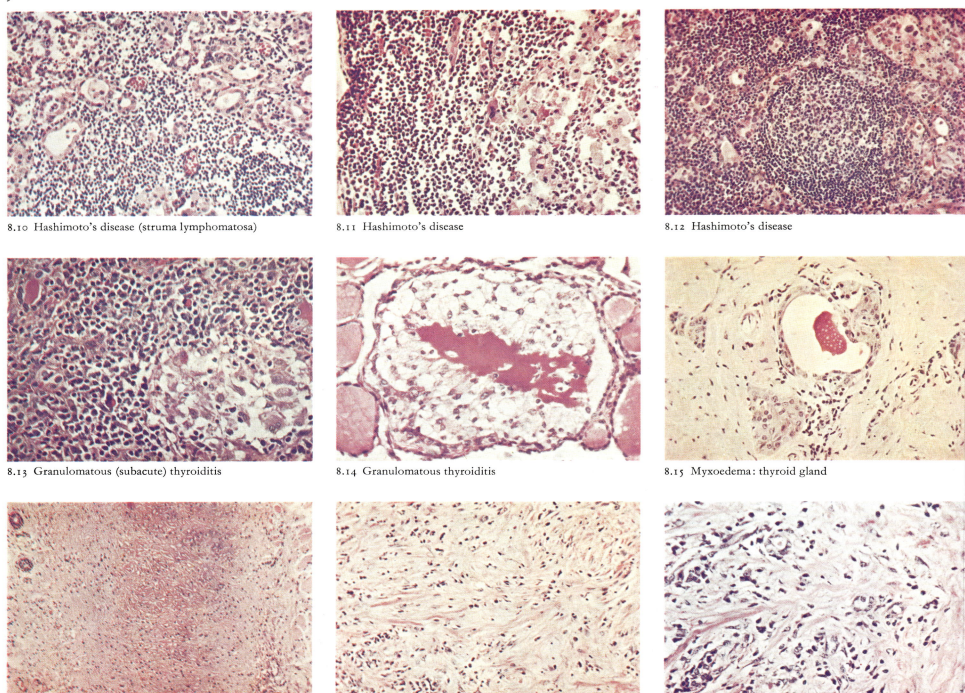

8.10 Hashimoto's disease (struma lymphomatosa)   8.11 Hashimoto's disease   8.12 Hashimoto's disease

8.13 Granulomatous (subacute) thyroiditis   8.14 Granulomatous thyroiditis   8.15 Myxoedema: thyroid gland

8.16 Myxoedema: vocal cord   8.17 Riedel's struma   8.18 Riedel's struma

8.10–8.12 Hashimoto's disease (struma lymphomatosa). 8.10 The epithelial cells are eosinophilic and form small irregular follicles which contain no colloid. The gland is heavily infiltrated with lymphocytes. **8.11** This is an area adjacent to that shown in 8.10 to show the distinctive large eosinophilic and pleomorphic epithelial (Askanazy) cells. These lie singly and in irregular groups among the numerous lymphocytes. **8.12** A lymphoid follicle with a germinal centre is present, and large numbers of lymphocytes lie between the follicles. Hashimoto's disease is an example of an auto-immune disease, the patients usually having a high titre of serum antibodies against thyroid colloid and epithelial cells. There is also evidence for an auto-immune process in its association with diseases such as pernicious (Addisonian) anaemia in which auto-antibody formation to gastric parietal cells occurs. **8.13 and 8.14 Granulomatous (subacute) thyroiditis.** This self-limiting disease may be of viral origin and is sometimes a complication of mumps. **8.13** Large numbers of lymphocytes and plasma cells have infiltrated between the follicles which are small and atrophic. Histiocytes have formed a small follicle (bottom right) similar to a tuberculous follicle. The lesion was focal. **8.14** Vacuolated phagocytes are attacking and breaking up

a mass of very dense colloid which appears to lie within a follicle. **8.15 Myxoedema: thyroid gland.** The gland was very small and firm. It consists of fibrous tissue and very scanty epithelial elements which form irregular groups and follicles. This follicle contains a small mass of dense vacuolated colloid. The atrophy of this gland was idiopathic. A fairly similar picture may follow therapy with radioactive iodine. Myxoedema may also develop in Hashimoto's disease. **8.16 Myxoedema: vocal cord.** Basophilic mucinous ground substance has been deposited (centre) in the vocal cord between the muscle (right) and the epithelium (left). The pale clefts in the material are occupied by connective tissue cells. **8.17 and 8.18 Riedel's struma.** The lesion was limited to one pole of the gland, which was adherent to surrounding structures in the neck. **8.17** The affected part consists of very dense fibrous tissue. There appear to be no epithelial cells, the pleomorphic nuclei apparently belonging to connective tissue cells. **8.18** Degenerate epithelial cells are present. They lie singly or form small very abnormal follicles. This condition is probably related to retroperitoneal and mediastinal fibrosis.

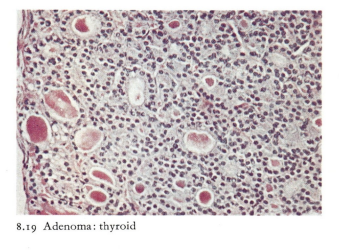

8.19 Adenoma: thyroid

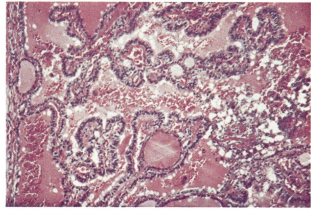

8.20 Primary papillary carcinoma: thyroid

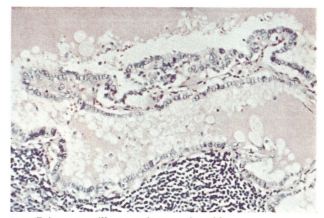

8.21 Primary papillary carcinoma: thyroid

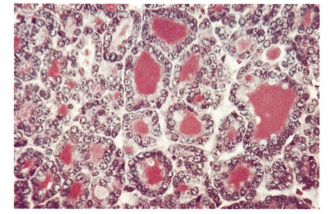

8.22 Primary follicular carcinoma: thyroid

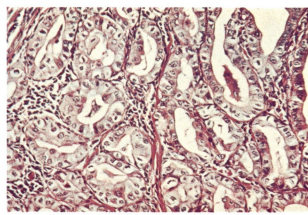

8.23 Primary follicular carcinoma: thyroid

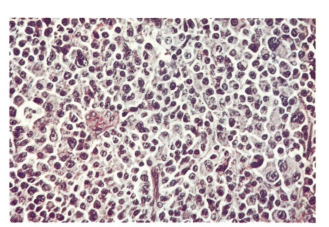

8.24 Primary undifferentiated carcinoma: thyroid

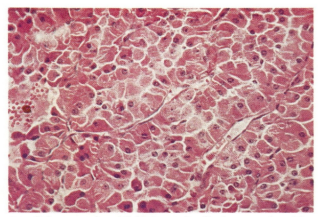

8.25 Primary eosinophil (Askanazy) cell adenoma: thyroid

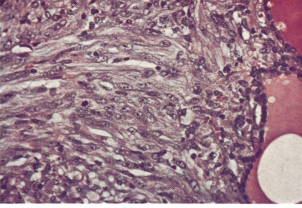

8.26 Primary sarcoma: thyroid

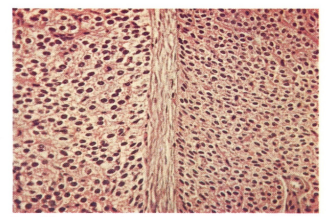

8.27 Adenoma: parathyroid

8.19 Adenoma: thyroid. This was a spherical mass completely enclosed in a fibrous capsule, part of which is visible here (left). The follicles are small and many have no lumen. The cells are cuboidal or columnar, but very regular in form and the nuclei show no mitotic activity. In endemic (iodine-deficiency) goitre, foci similar to this are found and to distinguish them from adenomas is virtually impossible. **8.20** and **8.21 Primary papillary carcinoma: thyroid. 8.20** Large papillary epithelial processes consisting of branching vascular stroma covered with cuboidal epithelium project into cystic follicular spaces which are full of colloid. The epithelial cells are very uniform and there are no mitoses. The papillary processes are much larger and more complex than in thyrotoxicosis. The tumour is a low-grade carcinoma but it may metastasize. **8.21** This is a secondary deposit in a lymph node of the tumour in 8.20. The tumour cells are cuboidal and very regular in form and no mitoses are present. They form a large cystic colloid-filled space into which a papilliform process projects. The lymphoid tissue is visible at the bottom. **8.22** and **8.23 Primary follicular carcinoma: thyroid.** This was a large tumour in a girl of 11 years who had had x-irradiation to her neck in infancy. It is well-differentiated. The epithelial cells are cuboidal with relatively large nuclei and form regular follicles mostly filled with dense colloid. There are scattered mitoses (top left, for example). The tumour was locally invasive and recurred several times. When a carcinoma of thyroid forms colloid like this, therapeutic administration of radioactive iodine (I131) is more likely to be beneficial since the isotope will

be incorporated in the colloid and have an opportunity to act more effectively on the epithelium. **8.23** This is a much more active tumour than 8.22. The cells are large and pleomorphic and form very irregular close-packed follicles. There is no colloid formation, but desquamated cells are present in some follicles. A slight papillary tendency is evident (top right). Lymphocytes are present in the fibrous stroma. **8.24 Primary undifferentiated carcinoma: thyroid.** The tumour is almost completely anaplastic and only one rudimentary follicle (centre left) is evident. The cells are fairly large and their pleomorphic nuclei have prominent nucleoli. Stroma is very scanty. Undifferentiated carcinomas may be confused with lymphosarcoma or reticulum cell sarcoma. **8.25 Eosinophil (Askanazy) cell adenoma: thyroid.** Macroscopically the tumour had a distinctive brown colour. The cells are characteristically large and have abundant eosinophilic cytoplasm. Their nuclei are regular but have prominent nucleoli. However, there are no mitotic figures. Stroma is very scanty. Askanazy cell tumours are generally benign. **8.26 Primary sarcoma: thyroid.** This is a spindle-cell tumour. The cells are large but form very little intercellular substance. There are many mitoses (left of centre, for example). **8.27 Adenoma: parathyroid.** Adenomas are generally solitary and produce primary hyperparathyroidism. The tumour is a solid mass of closely-packed polyhedral cells. The two groups of cells separated by a broad band of fibrous tissue stroma differ in size and degree of cytoplasmic eosinophilia (oxyphilia) but in both the cell size and nuclear form are fairly constant.

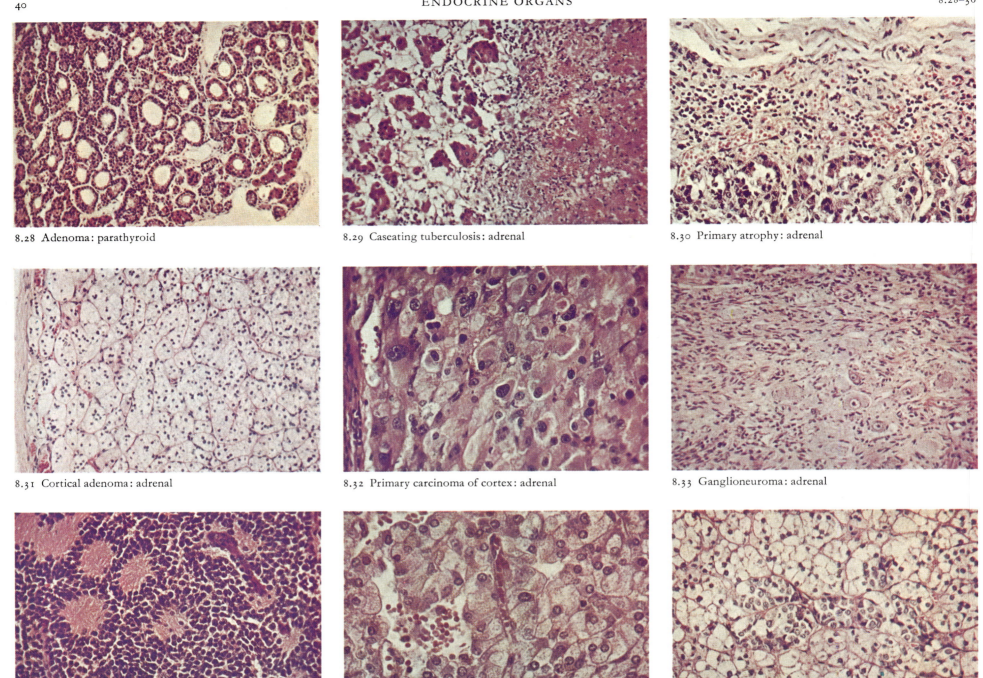

8.28 Adenoma: parathyroid

8.29 Caseating tuberculosis: adrenal

8.30 Primary atrophy: adrenal

8.31 Cortical adenoma: adrenal

8.32 Primary carcinoma of cortex: adrenal

8.33 Ganglioneuroma: adrenal

8.34 Neuroblastoma: adrenal

8.35 Phaeochromocytoma (chromaffinoma): adrenal

8.36 Secondary carcinoma: adrenal

8.28 Adenoma: parathyroid. In this tumour the cells are forming acini. Most cells are basophilic blue-staining chief cells but a few groups of oxyphil cells are present. The cells vary greatly in size and shape but the lesion is benign. Stroma is very scanty. Adenomas composed wholly of strongly oxyphil cells rarely cause hyperparathyroidism. **8.29 Caseating tuberculosis: adrenal.** This is generally secondary to pulmonary tuberculosis. The caseous tissue (right) is strongly eosinophilic and scattered throughout it are numerous nuclear fragments. On the left is one of the few small islands of cortical tissue that remained. The other adrenal gland was completely caseous and the patient had Addisons' disease. **8.30 Primary atrophy: adrenal.** This patient also died of Addison's disease. Loss of cortical tissue is complete, and between the fibrous tissue capsule (top) and the medulla (bottom) there are only dilated vascular spaces and an infiltrate of plasma cells and lymphocytes. Some patients with Addison's disease due to primary atrophy have antibodies to adrenal tissue in their serum and an auto-immune reaction has been postulated. **8.31 Cortical adenoma: adrenal.** The lesion was a spherical yellow mass 2 cm. in diameter and situated beneath the capsule (left) of the gland. Its cells are large and foamy (lipid-laden) and their arrangement is haphazard and unlike that of a normal gland. The nuclei are uniform and there are no mitoses. Many cortical adenomas exert no detectable endocrine effect. **8.32 Primary carcinoma of cortex: adrenal.** The tumour cells are large, have abundant granular cytoplasm and their nuclei are very pleomorphic. Some of the nuclei have very large nucleoli. Adrenocortical carcinomas sometimes exert hormonal effects. The capsule of the gland is on the left. **8.33 Ganglioneuroma: adrenal.** This rare benign tumour is composed of sympathetic ganglion cells and nerve fibres. It may arise elsewhere in the sympathetic nervous system. Tumours also occur which are a mixture of the benign ganglioneuroma and the more primitive and highly malignant neuroblastoma (ganglioneuroblastoma). **8.34 Neuroblastoma: adrenal.** This tumour was a secondary deposit in skeletal muscle. It consists of relatively small cells which have deeply basophilic nuclei and virtually no cytoplasm. The cells form circular 'rosettes' around a mass of very fine eosinophilic filaments. Stromal blood vessels are present on the right. **8.35 Phaeochromocytoma (chromaffinoma): adrenal.** The tumour is composed of mature cells which closely resemble those of the adrenal medulla. They possess abundant granular cytoplasm. The nuclei are uniform and the lesion is benign, though the cells line large vascular spaces. The stroma is very delicate. The cells secrete adrenaline and/or noradrenaline and produce the characteristic syndrome. If the tumour is fixed in bichromate solutions it turns brown ('chromaffin'). **8.36 Secondary carcinoma: adrenal.** This is a small deposit from an undifferentiated carcinoma of bronchus. The tumour cells are growing between the lipid-laden cells of the zona fasciculata. Small secondary deposits like this are not uncommon but are easily overlooked

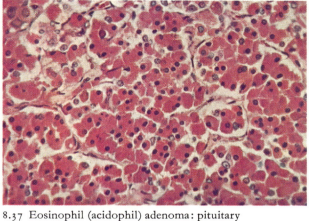

8.37 Eosinophil (acidophil) adenoma: pituitary

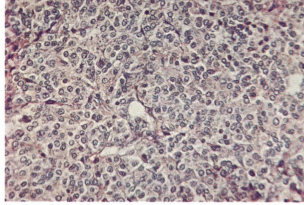

8.38 Chromophobe adenoma: pituitary

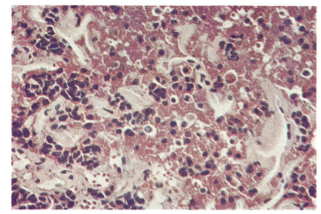

8.39 Secondary carcinoma: pituitary

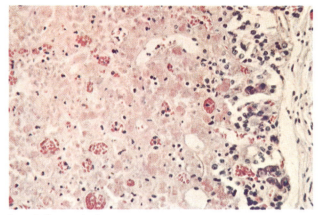

8.40 Infarct: pituitary

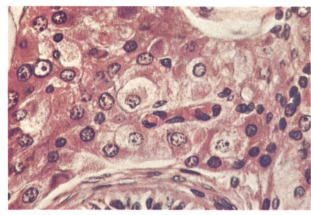

8.41 Klinefelter's syndrome: testis

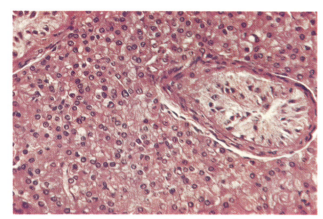

8.42 Hyperplasia of the interstitial cells: testis

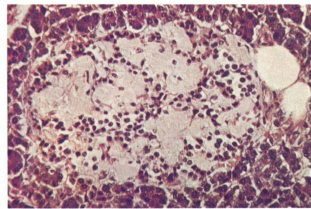

8.43 Diabetes mellitus: pancreatic islets

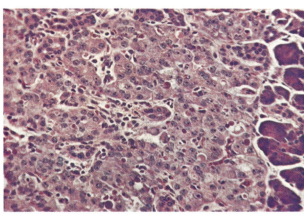

8.44 Adenoma: pancreatic islets

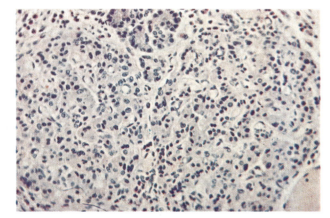

8.45 Hyperplasia: pancreatic islets

8.37 Eosinophil (acidophil) adenoma: pituitary. This was a well-defined mass 1 cm. in diameter. It consists of polygonal cells possessing abundant eosinophilic cytoplasm. A few chromophobe cells are present. This type of tumour produces gigantism and acromegaly. **8.38 Chromophobe adenoma: pituitary.** The cells have a moderate amount of cytoplasm which does not stain strongly with haematoxylin or eosin. The stroma is very scanty and delicate. Histologically these lesions look benign but they grow to a considerable size and exert important space-occupying effects, including destruction of active endocrine tissue in the rest of the gland. They are also invasive and penetrate the dural capsule of the gland to involve surrounding nervous and vascular structures. **8.39 Secondary carcinoma: pituitary.** The tumour cells (left) have pleomorphic and very basophilic nuclei but very little cytoplasm. The surrounding tissues are necrotic. This is part of the anterior pituitary, though secondary deposits are more common in the posterior pituitary. The primary growth was an undifferentiated ('oat-cell') carcinoma of lung. **8.40 Infarct: pituitary.** A thin layer of cells survives beneath the capsule of the gland (right). They are somewhat degenerate. The rest of the gland is necrotic. The sinusoids are dilated. A large infarct of the anterior pituitary causes Simmond's disease and may be produced by occlusion of either arteries or veins. Many cases of partial infarction result from an episode of hypotension following severe post-partum haemorrhage. The clinical picture is that of Sheehan's syndrome. **8.41 Klinefelter's syndrome: testis.** In this syndrome the patient is an abnormal infertile male with gynaecomastia and small testes and is often mentally defective. An extra X chromosome is present (XXY) in his cells. In this biopsy of testis, interstitial (Leydig) cells are numerous, and in some of the nuclei the extra X chromosome is manifest as a sex chromatin body, smaller than and quite distinct from the nucleolus (below the central capillary, for exam-

ple). At the bottom is part of a tubule with a thickened basement membrane. **8.42 Hyperplasia of the interstitial cells: testis.** There is very striking overgrowth of the interstitial cells and these fill the space between the tubules. This testis was undescended and the basement membrane of the tubules is thick and fibrous. Spermatogenesis is not taking place and the tubules contain only Sertoli cells. Interstitial cells form tumours that cause precocious physical and sexual development when present in young subjects. In adults they may cause gynaecomastia. **8.43 Diabetes mellitus: pancreatic islets.** Most of the islet tissue has been replaced by an amorphous hyaline material similar to amyloid. Hyalinisation of islets is seen in only a minority of diabetic subjects. Two fat cells are present (right) among the exocrine elements. **8.44 Adenoma: pancreatic islets.** The tumour cells resemble islet cells and are mainly arranged in anastomosing cords. However some form small clusters around a small lumen in which there is some eosinophilic material. The nuclei of the cells are very uniform but the nucleoli are very prominent. The tumour appears to be well-demarcated from the exocrine tissue (right) but there is no fibrous capsule and several small pancreatic ducts have been caught up in the tumour. There were no metastases. Most islet cell tumours are benign adenomas but there may be multiple growths in the pancreas. There may also be 'adenomas' in other endocrine glands. This patient suffered from hypoglycaemic episodes and presumably the cells are beta cells. Non-beta-cell adenomas may be associated with hypersecretion of acid and ulceration of duodenum and proximal jejunum (Zollinger-Ellison syndrome). **8.45 Hyperplasia: pancreatic islets.** This is the pancreas of an infant who died within a few hours of birth and whose mother was severely diabetic. It shows two of the many large and hyperplastic islets of Langerhans that were present. A small portion of exocrine tissue is visible (top).

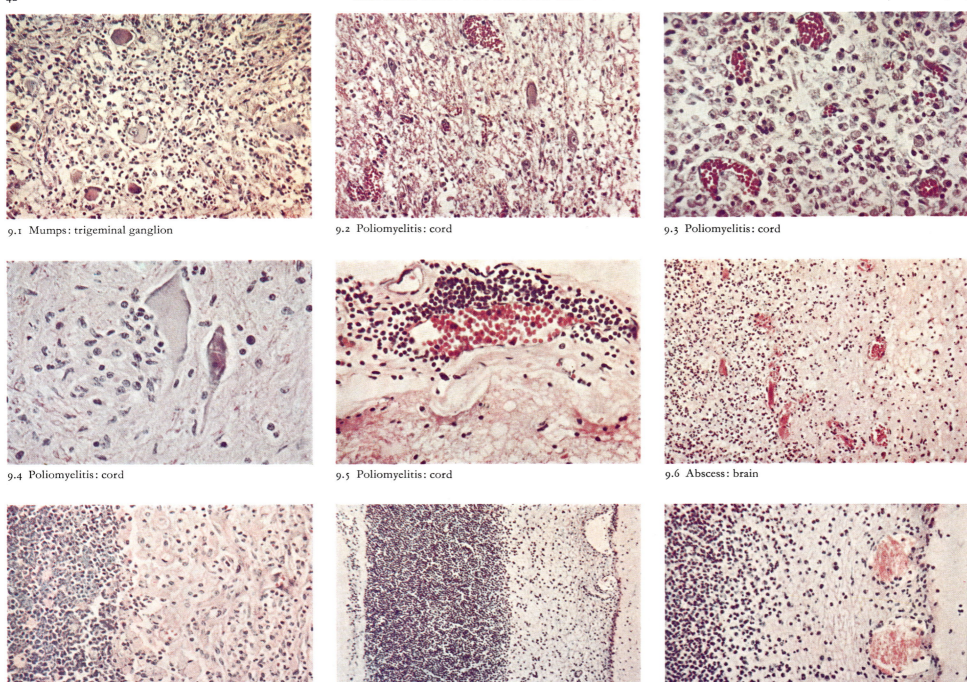

9.1 Mumps: trigeminal ganglion

9.2 Poliomyelitis: cord

9.3 Poliomyelitis: cord

9.4 Poliomyelitis: cord

9.5 Poliomyelitis: cord

9.6 Abscess: brain

9.7 Abscess: brain

9.8 Purulent meningitis

9.9 Purulent meningitis

9.1 Mumps: trigeminal ganglion. The ganglion has been almost completely destroyed and the neurons are in the various stages of degeneration. Lymphocytes and plasma cells are very numerous. There were no lesions in the brain and the patient died of myocardial and renal lesions. **9.2–9.5 Poliomyelitis. 9.2–9.4** The lesions are in the anterior horn of the spinal cord. **9.2** There has been very extensive destruction of neurons and only a few chromatolytic ones survive. The tissue is hyperaemic and oedematous. **9.3** Necrosis of neurons is complete here and only debris remains. Between the dilated capillaries are large numbers of lipid-laden microglial phagocytes (fat-granule cells or compound granular corpuscles). **9.4** The neurons are degenerate. One cell (left of centre) is undergoing neuronophagia. The cell right of centre is shrunken and shows ischaemic type degeneration. The hyperplastic microglial cells (left of centre) are almost certainly engaged in phagocytosing neuronal debris. **9.5** A small venule (top) is surrounded by lymphocytes in the subarachnoid space. The cord (bottom) is oedematous. **9.6** and **9.7 Abscess: brain. 9.6** This is the wall of an early abscess. The cerebral tissue is necrotic and heavily infiltrated with polymorphs (left). The capillaries are dilated and slight haemorrhage has

occurred. There is also oedema (right) at the periphery and the inflammatory process is extending into this, due to ineffective localization of infection in the cerebral white matter. **9.7** This lesion is more chronic than 9.6 The pus is out of the picture to the left. Next to it is a layer of necrotic cells and polymorphs (left) and external to this are lipid-laden microglial cells (centre) and elongated fibroblastic cells (right) which have already formed collagenous tissue (centre). **9.8** and **9.9 Purulent meningitis. 9.8** A purulent inflammatory exudate which consists largely of neutrophil polymorphs distends the subarachnoid space. Fibrin strands are fairly abundant. Inflammatory cells are also present in the arachnoid membrane (left) but the brain (right) itself is remarkably normal in appearance. **9.9** This is a high-power view of part of 9.8 and it shows that the exudate filling the subarachnoid space consists very largely of polymorphs and fibrin. The capillaries are very distended but the cortex (right) appears to be unaffected. A considerable proportion of these cases are caused by the pneumococcus.

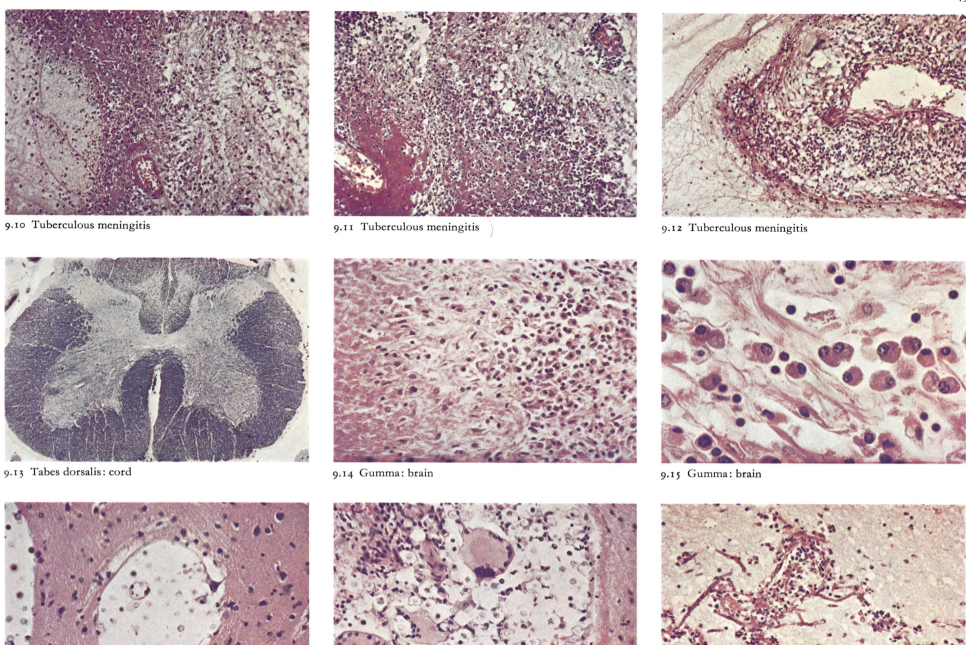

9.10   Tuberculous meningitis

9.11   Tuberculous meningitis

9.12   Tuberculous meningitis

9.13   Tabes dorsalis: cord

9.14   Gumma: brain

9.15   Gumma: brain

9.16   Cryptococcosis: brain

9.17   Cryptococcosis: brain

9.18   Aspergillosis: brain

9.10–9.12 Tuberculous meningitis. 9.10 The subarachnoid space (left) is full of inflammatory exudate. There are few viable cells in the exudate which consists largely of necrotic cellular debris and fibrin. The small vessel in the subarachnoid space is necrotic. The exudate is closely adherent to the cortex (right), which is severely oedematous and infiltrated by macrophages and lymphocytes. That is, there is a superficial encephalitis. **9.11** Damage to the cortex is more severe here. The vessel lying in the exudate in the subarachnoid space (bottom left) is necrotic and surrounded by densely stained fibrin. The cortex underlying the vessel (bottom right) is also necrotic. The adjacent tissue (top right) is very oedematous and inflammatory cells surround the small blood vessel. **9.12** The wall of a small cerebral artery lying in fibrinous exudate (left) in the subarachnoid space is inflamed. The intima is thickened and the media has been replaced by lymphocytes, epithelioid cells and giant cells. The lumen is much reduced, so that ischaemic effects are produced in the cortex, particularly if thrombosis supervenes. **9.13 Tabes dorsalis: cord.** The section through segment L4 of the spinal cord has been stained by the Loyez method for myelin. It shows the typical loss of large fibres in the middle root zone of the posterior columns (top centre). **9.14** and **9.15 Gumma: brain. 9.14** The necrotic centre of the gumma (left) is surrounded by macrophages and plasma cells. Some of the macrophages are epithelioid in form but there are no follicles. There is moderate fibrosis (centre). **9.15** In this part of the gumma

there are numerous plasma cells and a considerable amount of dense fibrous tissue. Each plasma cell has abundant dusky red cytoplasm and an eccentric nucleus in which the chromatin sometimes forms a 'cart-wheel' or 'clock-face' pattern. Lymphocytes are also present. **9.16** and **9.17 Cryptococcosis: brain. 9.16** In the cortex there are two typical 'soap-bubble' cysts (centre and left) full of the organism, *Cryptococcus neoformans* (*Torula histolytica*). Only the centre of the organism is visible, the thick gelatinous capsule remaining unstained. These cysts generally communicate through a narrow opening with the subarachnoid space. **9.17** This shows another cyst in the superficial cortex which contains large numbers of the organism. There is relatively little microglial or macroglial reaction in the underlying cortex (right) but in the subarachnoid space (left) there is fibroplasia and giant-cell formation. As in 9.16 the organism stains very lightly and its thick capsule is completely colourless. **9.18 Aspergillosis: brain.** The branching tubular filamentous organism is growing in the brain in the vicinity of a small venule and several capillaries. Polymorphs are numerous in and around the vessels but there appears to be very little reaction to the filaments of the organism as they spread outwards. The patient was a girl of 13 who had Hodgkin's disease and was treated with chemotherapy including nitrogen mustard and chlorambucil.

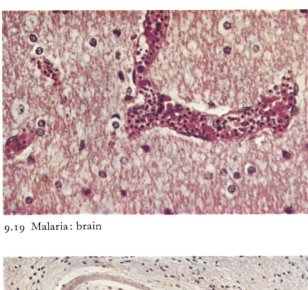

9.19 Malaria: brain

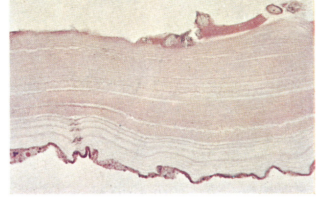

9.20 Hydatid disease (echinococcosis): brain

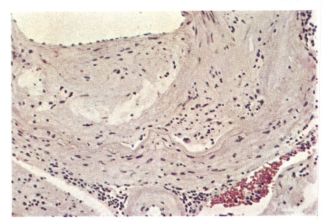

9.21 Atherosclerosis: cerebral artery

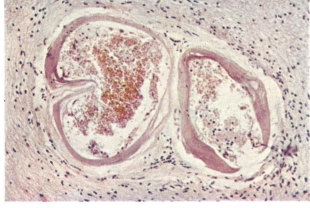

9.22 Arteriosclerosis: cerebral artery

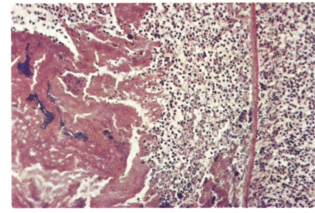

9.23 Mycotic aneurysm: cerebral artery

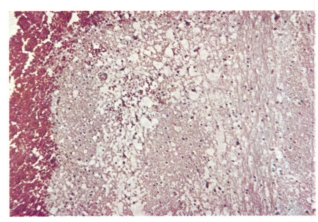

9.24 Cerebral haemorrhage

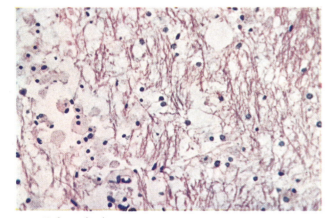

9.25 Infarct: brain

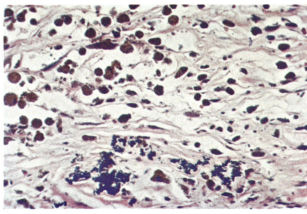

9.26 Infarct: brain

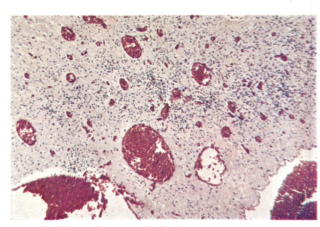

9.27 Capillary telangiectasis: brain

9.19 Malaria: brain. The capillaries are engorged and a high proportion of the erythrocytes contain the parasite (P. falciparum). The oligodendrocytes show the characteristic perinuclear space. **9.20 Hydatid disease (echinococcosis): brain.** The cyst was unilocular and this shows the cuticular or laminated layer which consists of acellular chitin. **9.21 Atherosclerosis: cerebral artery.** The media of this small artery is thin and fibrous, with considerable loss of muscle cells. The internal elastic lamina is split and frayed and a crescentic mass of tissue (top left) partly fills the lumen. The tissue consists of loose connective tissue in which abundant lipid could be demonstrated in frozen sections. Lymphocytes are also present. Endothelium covers the plaque. The arteriole (bottom centre) shows severe sclerotic changes and its lumen is considerably narrowed. **9.22 Arteriosclerosis: cerebral artery.** This is a small cerebral artery whose muscular wall is completely degenerate, consisting of hyaline fibrous tissue. The break in the wall (bottom right) is artefactual but the ease with which such a vessel may rupture is readily appreciated. **9.23 Mycotic aneurysm: cerebral artery.** The patient had subacute bacterial endocarditis. The wall of this small artery has been almost completely destroyed and shows aneurysmal dilatation. It is intensely infiltrated with polymorphs and macrophages and only a very thin layer of degenerate muscle (right) remains. The dilated lumen is full of thrombus (centre and left) which is largely fibrinous and in which colonies of bacteria (deep blue) are

growing. At the periphery of the thrombus there are many polymorphs (right of centre). **9.24 Cerebral haemorrhage.** The haemorrhage is in the globus pallidus and this is the edge (left). The brain adjacent to the haemorrhage (centre and right) is necrotic and oedematous. The round basophilic bodies are ischaemic nerve cells and some nerve cells and glial cells have disappeared. **9.25 and 9.26 Infarct: brain. 9.25** This is the edge of an infarct of about six weeks' duration. The cerebral white matter has a spongy texture due to the ischaemic necrosis of many myelinated fibres. Foamy (lipid-laden) microglial cells (fat-granule cells or compound granular corpuscles) are present (left mainly) in the interstices of surviving fibres. A number of astrocytes, some hypertrophic, are present. The spaces were filled with watery fluid. **9.26** This is an old infarct which appeared as a yellowish plaque during post-mortem examination. It consists of dense collagenous tissue, though the scar in healed lesions is usually mostly neuroglial. Part of the fibrous tissue has calcified (bottom), and throughout it there are numerous haemosiderin-laden phagocytes (microglia). **9.27 Capillary telangiectasis: brain.** The lesion, which was solitary, consists of abnormally dilated capillaries of widely varying calibre. The vessels are separated by neural tissue. There is no evidence of previous haemorrhage. In contrast the vessels in cavernous angiomas are contiguous, usually thick-walled, and liable to rupture.

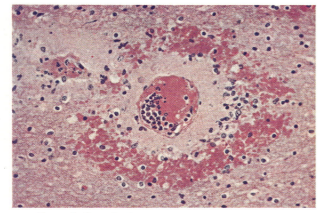

9.28 Fat embolism: brain

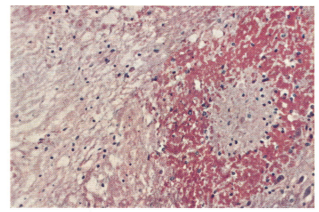

9.29 Fat embolism: brain

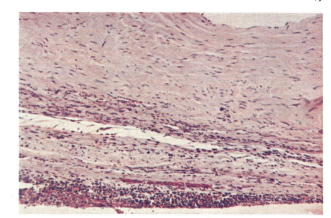

9.30 Chronic subdural haematoma
(pachymeningitis haemorrhagica interna)

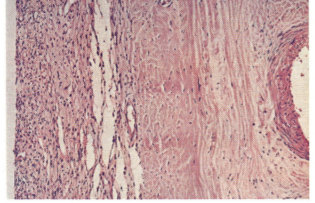

9.31 Chronic subdural haematoma

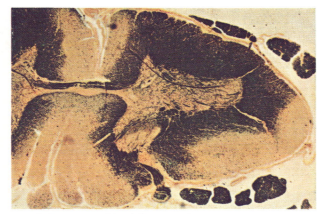

9.32 Subacute combined degeneration: cord

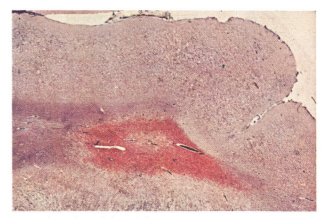

9.33 Disseminated (multiple) sclerosis: brain

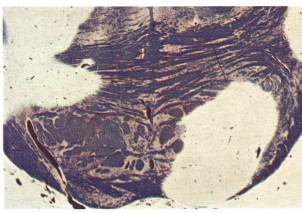

9.34 Disseminated sclerosis: brain

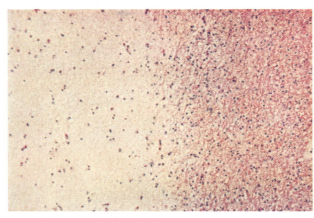

9.35 Disseminated sclerosis: brain

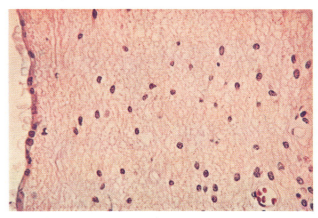

9.36 Disseminated sclerosis: brain

9.28 and **9.29 Fat embolism: brain. 9.28** The arteriole (centre) is plugged with conglutinated red cells and polymorphs. The cerebral tissue around the vessel is necrotic and there is haemorrhage. Microglial cells are proliferating at the inner margin of the haemorrhage. A frozen section showed a considerable amount of fat in the lumen of many arterioles and capillaries. The origin of the fat was a fracture of femur. **9.29** There is a small ring haemorrhage (right) with ischaemia and oedema of the adjacent white matter (left). A neuron in the haemorrhage shows ischaemic change. **9.30** and **9.31 Chronic subdural haematoma (pachymeningitis haemorrhagica interna). 9.30** The dura occupies the top half of the picture. There has been haemorrhage from the superficial cerebral veins in the subdural space and this blood has been organised to form a layer of fibrous tissue on the inner surface of the dura. On the free (arachnoidal) surface of this new tissue (bottom) where fibroplasia is characteristically tardy an area of organising haemorrhage is still visible. **9.31** Here the densely fibrous dura occupies the centre and right parts of the picture. In its inner surface (left) a layer of connective tissue has formed in which there are thin-walled blood vessels from which further haemorrhage and serous exudation readily occurs. This tissue, which is still fairly cellular and contains many macrophages, was not adherent to the arachnoid. A small artery is present on the right. A subdural haematoma is a space-occupying lesion and though generally thought to be traumatic in origin, is sometimes associated with blood dyscrasias. **9.32 Subacute combined degeneration.** This is a section of the spinal cord (C5) stained by the Weigert-Pal method for myelin. The nerve roots are unaffected but the following tracts are degenerate: the posterior columns (gracilis and part of cuneate) (bottom left); the anterior (direct) cerebrospinal (top left); and the anterior and posterior spinocerebellar and lateral (crossed) cerebrospinal tract (below right). **9.33–9.36 Disseminated (multiple) sclerosis. 9.33** This is a frozen section of cerebrum stained with Sudan IV to show fat. In the central white matter it shows a recent lesion in which much stainable fat is present (below centre). The fat comes from the breakdown of the complex lipids of the myelin of the medullary sheaths. Above and to the left of the lesion, the subcortical 'U' fibres (blue-staining) have been spared. **9.34** The section of mid-pons has been stained by the Loyez method for myelin. There are three large lesions in which loss of myelin is complete. Note the random distribution of the plaques. **9.35** The plaque (left) shows pallor due to loss of myelin. The cells within it are few in number and mostly astrocytes. Compare with the adjoining normal white matter (right) where oligodendroglial cells are numerous. **9.36** This is an old periventricular plaque which consists entirely of astrocytes and glial fibres. The pale blue body (left of centre) is a calcospherite. The ependymal lining of the ventricle is visible on the left.

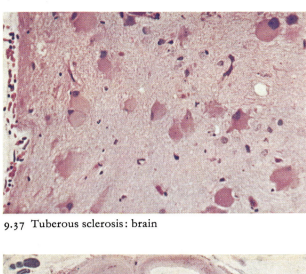

9.37 Tuberous sclerosis: brain

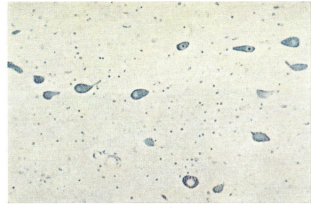

9.38 Motor neuron disease (progressive muscular atrophy): cord

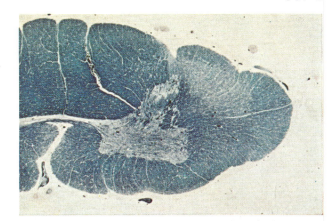

9.39 Motor neuron disease (amyotrophic lateral sclerosis): cord

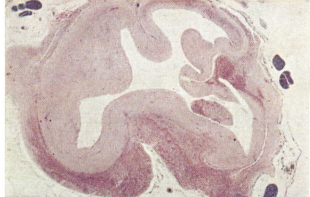

9.40 Syringomyelia: cord

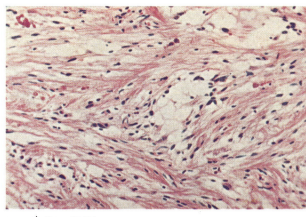

9.41 Astrocytoma

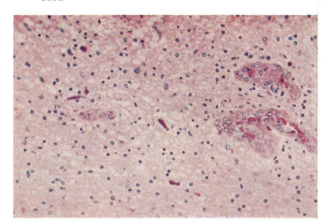

9.42 Astrocytoma

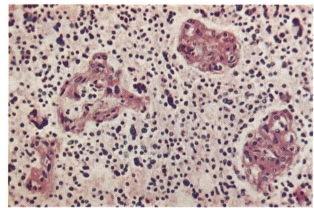

9.43 Astrocytoma

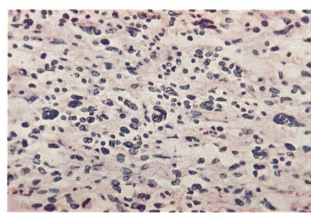

9.44 Astrocytoma

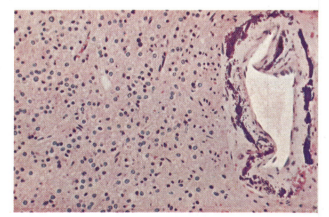

9.45 Oligodendrocytoma

9.37 Tuberous sclerosis. This is the cerebral cortex. The normal architecture is absent and the tissue consists of abundant glial fibrils in which there are numerous bizarre giant cells. These abnormal cells are characteristic of this condition and some have features of neurons and others of astrocytes. This condition is generally associated with sebaceous adenomas of the skin and hamartomas of the kidney, as well as with mental deficiency. **9.38 Motor neuron disease (progressive muscular atrophy).** This section of the spinal cord has been stained with thionin to show the motor neurons in the anterior horn. There are far fewer neurons than normal and the remaining cells show evidence of karyolysis (top left) and chromatolysis (centre and far right of centre, for example). Degeneration of anterior horn cells leads to muscular atrophy. **9.39 Motor neuron disease (amyotrophic lateral sclerosis).** This section of cord has been stained by the Loyez method for myelin. There is atrophy of the cerebrospinal (pyramidal) tracts which is revealed as pallor due to loss of myelinated fibres throughout the lateral and anterior columns. The change is more pronounced in the crossed cerebrospinal tract (above and right of centre) than in the direct tract (below left). Degeneration of the pyramidal tracts produces spastic paralysis. Later in this syndrome there is degeneration of anterior horn neurons and muscular changes similar to progressive muscular atrophy. **9.40 Syringomyelia.** This is the spinal cord at the level of C7. The central portion of the cord is occupied by a cystic structure, now partially collapsed, which greatly distorts and has caused atrophy of the neural tissue. The cyst is lined by dense glial tissue. Classically there is loss of the senses of pain and temperature

and preservation of those for pressure and touch. **9.41–9.44 Astrocytoma.** 9.41 and 9.42 are fairly well-differentiated lesions (Grades 1 or 2). **9.41** In this tumour the fibrillary processes of the mature astrocytes are prominent and there is also considerable fluid in their interstices, with formation of many microcysts. Strongly eosinophilic Rosenthal fibres are present in some of the cells. These are not specific for astrocytomas but may be found in reactive gliosis. **9.42** The neoplastic astrocytes show moderate pleomorphism. The capillaries are tortuous and the endothelial cells are hyperplastic and hypertrophied. This change in the capillaries is often most marked at the edge of the tumour and is particularly pronounced in those of Grades 3 and 4. **9.43** and **9.44** These two tumours are more malignant and are therefore classifiable as Grade 3 or 4 astrocytomas. In the older terminology they would be called glioblastoma multiforme. Both show great pleomorphism of the poorly differentiated astrocytes. The cells vary greatly in size and shape and there are many giant and multinucleate forms. In 9.43 the endothelial cells of the capillaries have proliferated greatly to form prominent buds with resultant reduction in their lumen. Necrosis was present in both tumours. In 9.44 a mitotic figure is visible (bottom left). **9.45 Oligodendrocytoma.** Though slow-growing, this tumour is highly cellular. Each cell has a small round nucleus round which there is a clear zone or halo; 'boxing' of the nucleus. Calcium deposition, which is a frequent occurrence in this type of tumour, is present in the media of a small vessel (right).

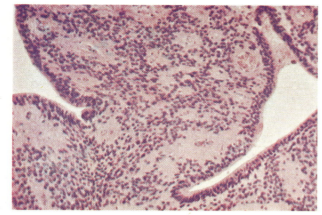

9.46 Ependymoma

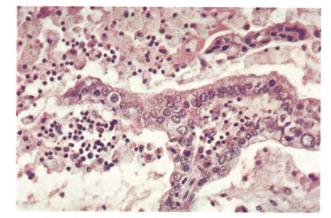

9.47 Secondary carcinoma: brain

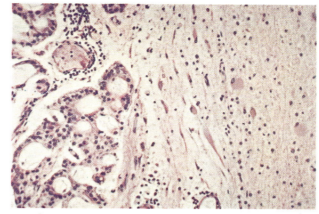

9.48 Secondary carcinoma: brain

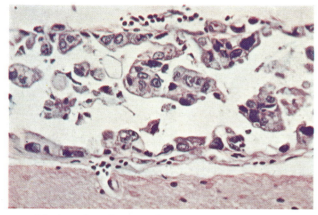

9.49 Meningeal carcinomatosis

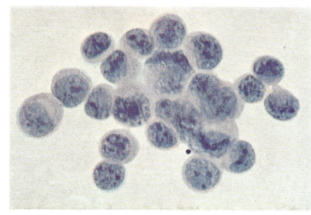

9.50 Carcinoma cells: cerebrospinal fluid

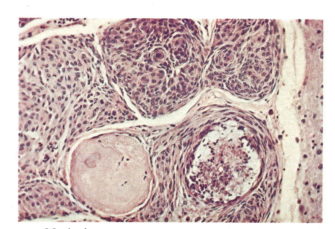

9.51 Meningioma

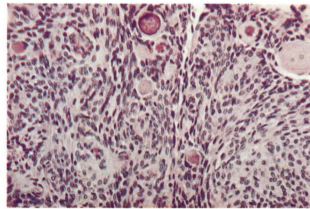

9.52 Meningioma

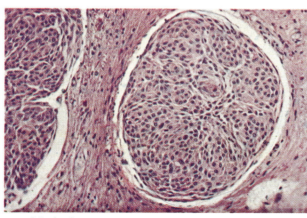

9.53 Meningioma

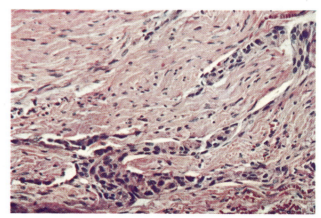

9.54 Meningioma

9.46 Ependymoma. This tumour is derived from the ependymal cells lining the ventricles and central canal. It is a cellular neoplasm intersected by channels, lined by columnar cells, which resemble central canals. The structure here is mainly that of the 'epithelial' form of ependymoma. The cells between the canals are also ependymal and some of them form characteristic perivascular pseudorosettes which consist of radiating fibrillary processes. **9.47 and 9.48 Secondary carcinoma: brain. 9.47** This is a secondary from a carcinoma of breast. It is a papillary adenocarcinoma consisting of tall columnar epithelial cells clothing a delicate stroma. Mitotic activity is marked in the epithelium. Lymphocytes are present in and around the tumour, and there are many foamy (lipid-laden) microglial cells (top). There is considerable oedema. **9.48** This secondary deposit (left) in the cerebrum is from an adenocarcinoma of bronchus. The adjacent white matter (right) is oedematous and shows loosening of texture. Some astrocytes (bottom right) show early hyperplasia and some are swollen and hypertrophied. These changes are characteristic of cerebral oedema. **9.49 Meningeal carcinomatosis.** Tumour cells are growing freely in the subarachnoid space. They show great variation in structure, particularly in the nucleus. A few are shrunken and necrotic. The pia and cortex are visible at the bottom and a few lymphocytes are visible. The primary was a carcinoma of bronchus. **9.50 Carcinoma cells: cerebro-**

spinal fluid. This is a smear of the sediment from the cerebrospinal fluid, stained with methylene blue. The cells are large and form clumps. The nuclei are large and pleomorphic and have one or more nucleoli. The cytoplasm is pale-staining and scanty. The primary tumour was an undifferentiated carcinoma of the bronchus. **9.51–9.54 Meningioma. 9.51** The tumour is composed of large cells of arachnoidal type which show a marked tendency to a concentric whorled arrangement ('meningothelioma'). The centres of some of these whorls are becoming hyalinised and one forms a large hyaline body (bottom left). The cells at the periphery of the whorls are very flat, elongated and 'fibroblastic'. Nevertheless they do not form collagen. Some meningiomas are composed entirely of cells of this type. Tumour has not transgressed the pia mater and though the cerebral cortex (right) is being compressed it has not been invaded. **9.52** This tumour, similar in structure to 9.51, is noteworthy for the presence of many hyalinised and calcified foci (psammoma bodies). The lack of a distinct boundary between the tumour cells is evident. **9.53** From the main mass of tumour on the left a finger-like growth (right) has penetrated into the white matter, which is compressed and degenerating. **9.54** Like 9.53 this demonstrates the locally invasive powers of meningiomas. It shows tumour cells permeating the tissue spaces in the densely fibrous dura mater.

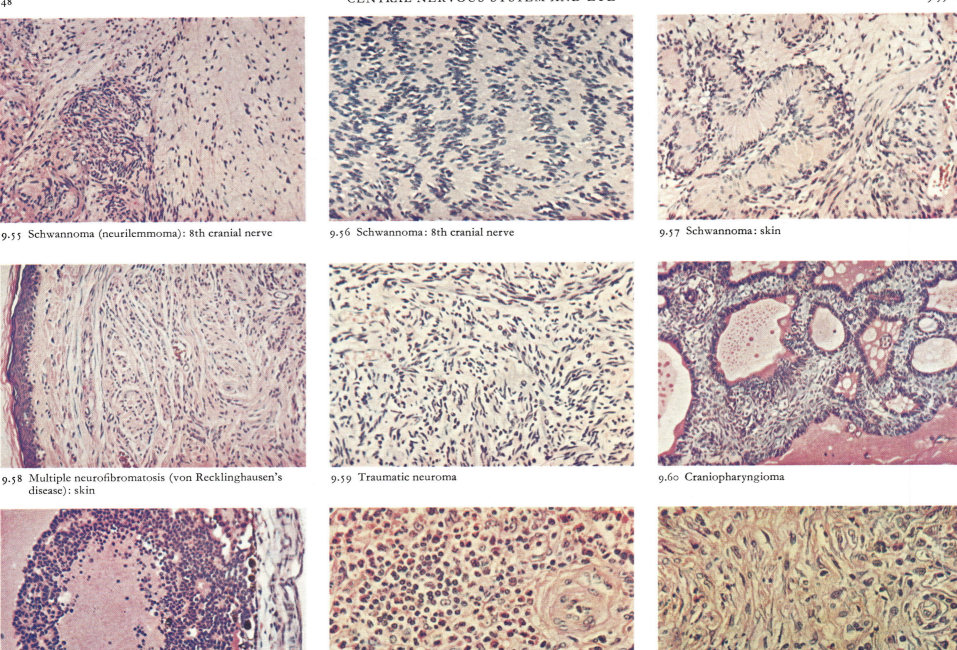

9.55 Schwannoma (neurilemmoma): 8th cranial nerve

9.56 Schwannoma: 8th cranial nerve

9.57 Schwannoma: skin

9.58 Multiple neurofibromatosis (von Recklinghausen's disease): skin

9.59 Traumatic neuroma

9.60 Craniopharyngioma

9.61 Retinoblastoma

9.62 Chronic granuloma (pseudotumour): orbit

9.63 Chronic granuloma: orbit

9.55–9.57 Schwannoma (neurilemmoma). 9.55 and **9.56** have arisen from Schwann cells in the auditory (8th cranial) nerve (acoustic neuromas). **9.55** Two types of tissue are present: compact interlacing networks of cells (lower left) (Antoni type A tissue) and a loose somewhat myxoid reticular tissue (right) (Antoni type B tissue) in which there are many spaces. Most of these contained watery fluid. Very little collagen could be demonstrated in the lesion. **9.56** Here the Schwann cells nuclei are arranged in parallel rows (palisading). The eosinophilic intercellular material appears fibrillary but very little collagen was present. **9.57** This tumour was in the subcutaneous tissues. The palisade arrangement of the Schwann cell nuclei is striking. The small amount of loose reticular (type B) tissue in this section is showing early degeneration and a tendency to cyst formation. **9.58 Multiple neurofibromatosis (von Recklinghausen's disease).** This is one of the multiple skin lesions. The tumour cells are more fibroblastic than the Schwann cells of the neurilemmoma and a considerable amount of stainable collagen in well-defined bundles can usually by demonstrated. Nerve fibres are generally also present. Neurofibromas in von Recklinghausen's disease are non-encapsulated and may become malignant. The overlying epidermis contains an excessive number of melanocytes ('café-au-lait') and pigment-laden macrophages are present in the dermis. **9.59 Traumatic neuroma.** These lesions are the result of trauma, often an amputation. They consist of proliferated Schwann cells lying in a very delicate connective tissue. This tends later to become collagenous and a certain amount of collagen could be demonstrated in this lesion. Large numbers of neurofibrils can also be invariably demonstrated. **9.60 Craniopharyngioma.** Columnar epithelial cells which resemble basal cells line small cystic spaces, some containing eosinophilic fluid. There is abundant loose connective tissue stroma. This combination of columnar cells and stroma which resembles a stellate reticulum accounts for use of the term 'adamantinoma' to describe this form of lesion. The epithelium is in fact often squamous. Craniopharyngiomas are believed to arise from displaced remnants of the embryonic hypophysial duct. They are nearly always suprasellar. This tumour was found in the region of the pituitary stalk. **9.61 Retinoblastoma.** This is a tumour of early childhood. The tumour covers the inner surface of the retina (right) and is invading the vitreous humour (left). The cells are very uniform, each possessing a large basophilic nucleus but no visible cytoplasm. They form many rosettes, the eosinophilic central part of which consists of fine fibrils. Some rosettes have a small blood vessel at the centre ('pseudorosettes'). Isolated cells are floating in the vitreous and some of these may 'seed' and grow on the adjacent retina. The medulloblastoma has a very similar structure. **9.62** and **9.63 Chronic granuloma (pseudotumour): orbit.** This lesion can behave like a neoplasm, forming a firm, localised mass which enlarges rapidly and causes exophthalmos. **9.62** This part of the lesion is cellular and there is only early fibrosis. The cells are mainly eosinophil polymorphs and lymphocytes but a few macrophages and plasma cells are evident. The appearances might be confused with eosinophilic granuloma or Hodgkin's disease. The 'onion-skin' thickening of the adventitia of the small artery (right), though a non-specific inflammatory response, is reminiscent of the changes that affect small arteries in the spleen in systemic lupus erythematosus. **9.63** Fibrous tissue formation is predominant. It tends to be centred round blood vessels, a blood vessel being out of the picture to the left. However, besides the fibroblasts there is a considerable population of macrophages, plasma cells, lymphocytes and eosinophils.

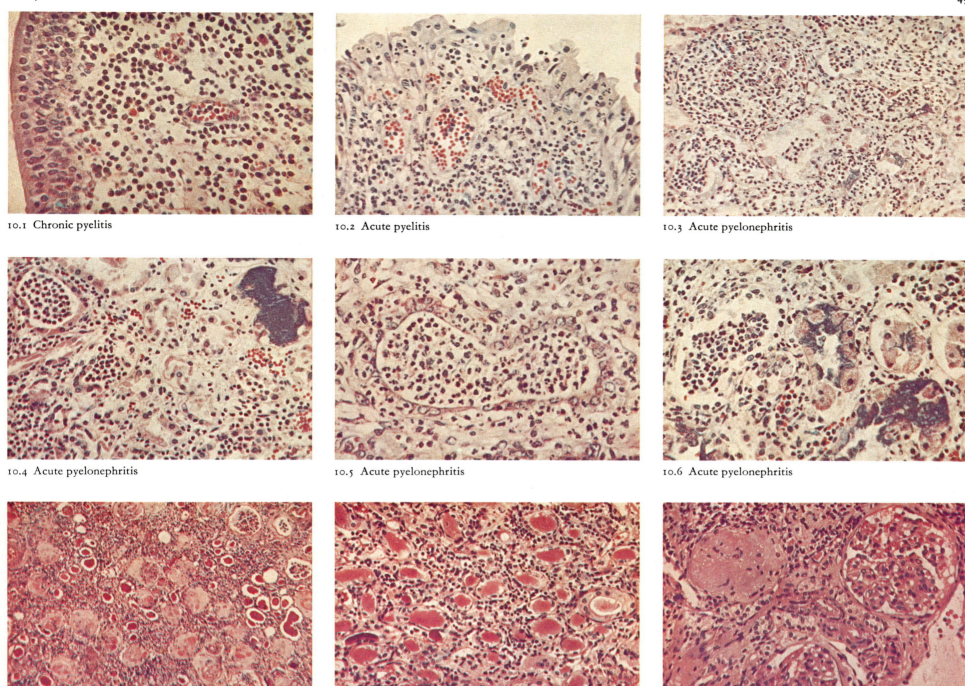

10.1 Chronic pyelitis

10.2 Acute pyelitis

10.3 Acute pyelonephritis

10.4 Acute pyelonephritis

10.5 Acute pyelonephritis

10.6 Acute pyelonephritis

10.7 Chronic pyelonephritis

10.8 Chronic pyelonephritis

10.9 Chronic pyelonephritis

10.1 Chronic pyelitis. The tissues are oedematous and hyperaemic and many inflammatory cells, nearly all plasma cells, are present beneath transitional epithelium (left). A few polymorphs are migrating through the epithelium to the lumen of the renal pelvis. **10.2 Acute pyelitis.** Here the ureter is more acutely inflamed. Hyperaemia is even more pronounced and many of the inflammatory cells are polymorphs. These lie in the sub-epithelial tissue between the dilated capillaries and some are penetrating the oedematous transitional epithelium to the lumen (above). Some mononuclear cells (lymphocytes and macrophages) are also present. It is rare for the renal pelvis alone to be inflamed and the kidney is usually also affected. **10.3–10.6 Acute pyelonephritis.** The patient had a carcinoma of prostate and developed 'ascending' pyelonephritis. **10.3** The convoluted tubules are filled with polymorphs and their epithelium is degenerate. Blue granular clumps of bacteria can also be identified in some tubules. Polymorphs also infiltrate the interstitial connective tissues and fill the subcapsular space of the glomerulus (top left) causing the tuft to shrink. **10.4** Some of the secretory tubules are filled with polymorphs and some with bacteria (top right). The stroma is oedematous and lightly infiltrated with inflammatory cells. The capillaries are very congested. **10.5** The collecting tubule is full of pus which here consists largely of polymorphs and fibrin. Polymorphs are also migrating through the degenerate epithelium lining the tubule. There is great oedema and leucocytic infiltration of the interstitial

tissue. **10.6** The epithelium lining some of the convoluted tubules (right) is swollen, eosinophilic and granular (cloudy swelling). Large numbers of bacteria (deep blue) are growing between these cells and in the lumen, and the cells are tending to disintegrate. This is more marked in the pus-filled tubule on the left where many of the cells have already sloughed off. Inflammatory cells are also infiltrating the stromal connective tissues around the tubules. **10.7–10.9 Chronic pyelonephritis. 10.7** The glomeruli are nearly all fibrosed and avascular. There is great tubular atrophy and the relatively few tubules that remain are dilated and contain densely eosinophilic ('colloid') casts. The interstitial tissue is extensively infiltrated with chronic inflammatory cells (lymphocytes and plasma cells). **10.8** This higher-power view shows the marked resemblance of the dense casts in the collecting tubules to thyroid colloid. The interstitial tissues are heavily infiltrated with lymphocytes. **10.9** One glomerulus (top right) looks more or less normal though Bowman's capsule is slightly thickened. Another (bottom centre) is atrophic and adherent to Bowman's capsule. The third (top left) is completely hyalinised, fibrous and avascular. Tubules of the loop of Henle survive around the less affected glomeruli. The interstitial tissue contains many lymphocytes. The histological picture of advanced chronic pyelonephritis may be very similar to that in advanced glomerulonephritis and when the pyelonephritic changes are diffuse and bilateral, macroscopic differentiation may be very difficult too.

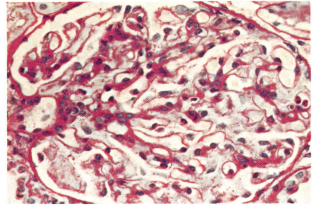

10.10 'Minimal change' glomerulonephritis

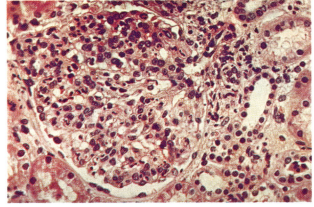

10.11 Acute proliferative glomerulonephritis

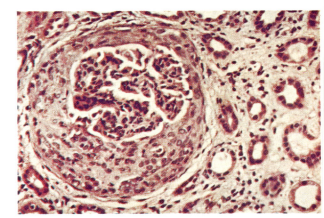

10.12 Proliferative glomerulonephritis with crescents

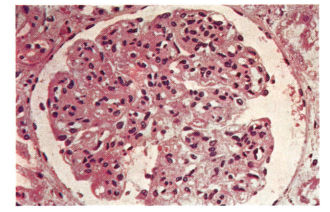

10.13 Membrano-proliferative glomerulonephritis

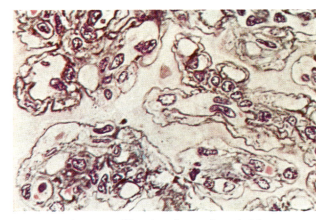

10.14 Membrano-proliferative glomerulonephritis

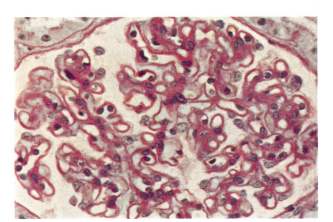

10.15 Membranous glomerulonephritis

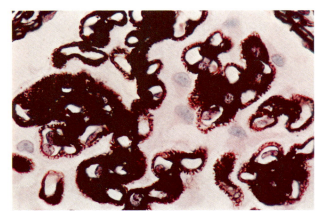

10.16 Membranous glomerulonephritis

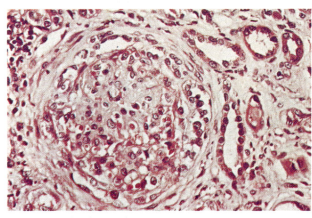

10.17 Chronic glomerulonephritis

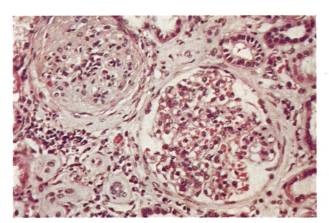

10.18 Chronic glomerulonephritis

10.10 'Minimal change' glomerulonephritis. Although this specimen was taken from a patient suffering from nephrotic syndrome with a heavy proteinuria, the glomerulus shows no significant abnormality, even when stained (as here) by the periodic acid-Schiff (PAS) method. In particular there is no cellular proliferation and no thickening of the glomerular basement membrane. The amount of PAS-positive (magenta-coloured) material at the centres of the glomerular lobules is within the normal range of variation. **10.11 Acute proliferative glomerulonephritis.** The glomerular tuft shows a marked increase in cellularity due to proliferation of endothelial cells and to infiltration with polymorphs. The increased number of swollen endothelial cells has obliterated the lumen of many capillaries, and the swollen tuft has almost obliterated Bowman's space. There is oedema of the interstitial tissues separating the tubules. **10.12 Proliferative glomerulonephritis with crescents.** In this form of proliferative glomerulonephritis, the glomerular epithelial cells proliferate. In this example, they have proliferated to such an extent as to form a large cellular 'crescent' which fills Bowman's space and compresses the glomerulus. The adjacent tubules are widely separated from one another by oedematous interstitial tissue. The normal epithelium of the tubules is replaced by a low simple epithelium, possibly due to regeneration following previous tubular damage. **10.13 and 10.14 Membrano-proliferative glomerulonephritis.** This is a special form of endothelial cell proliferative glomerulonephritis which commonly follows a slowly progressive course over several years. **10.13** Throughout the tuft there is an increase in endothelial cells and also a diffuse eosinophilic sclerosis. **10.14** In this thin (0.5 μm) section stained by the periodic acid-methenamine silver method it is possible to see the changes more clearly. Several capillaries are shown and the increase in endothelial cells is evident in the number of nuclei visible. The sclerosis can be seen to be due to formation of fine black-staining fibres and in some areas, e.g. in the capillary tuft

to the right of the centre, the glomerular basement membrane appears as a double line as a result of new fibres being laid down within the pre-existing glomerular basement membrane. **10.15 and 10.16 Membranous glomerulonephritis. 10.15** This PAS-stained section shows the characteristic lesion to consist of a diffuse thickening of the basement membrane. There is no proliferation of cells. The diffuse nature of the thickening, in that every capillary within the tuft is affected almost equally, is typical. Compare with 10.10. **10.16** It is occasionally difficult in ordinary preparations to distinguish between membranous and membrano-proliferative glomerulonephritis and the changes found in thin (0.5 μm) sections stained by the PA-methenamine silver method are then helpful. In the several capillaries shown here, the changes typical of membranous glomerulonephritis are evident: the glomerular basement membrane is seen to consist of an inner continuous black line with stumpy black 'bristles' on its outer surface. Compare with 10.14. **10.17 and 10.18 Chronic glomerulonephritis. 10.17** The glomerular tuft is sclerosed and many of its capillaries are obliterated. There are extensive capsular adhesions reducing Bowman's space to several narrow slits that are lined by proliferated, somewhat enlarged, epithelial cells. There is marked periglomerular and interstitial fibrosis. The tubules on the right are so damaged that it is not possible to identify them with certainly but they are probably grossly altered proximal convoluted tubules. **10.18** One glomerular tuft (right) appears relatively normal, but it is lightly adherent in several places to Bowman's capsule which itself is fibrosed. Its tubules survive but the epithelium of the convoluted tubules (right) is flat and degenerate. The other glomerulus (top left) is sclerosed and practically avascular. The subcapsular space is obliterated and Bowman's capsule is thick and fibrous. The interstitial tissue is fibrous and infiltrated with lymphocytes. There are hyalinised arterioles (bottom left).

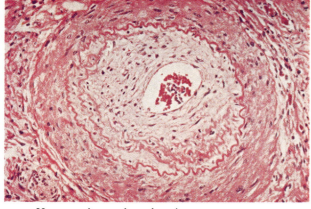

10.19 Hypertensive nephrosclerosis

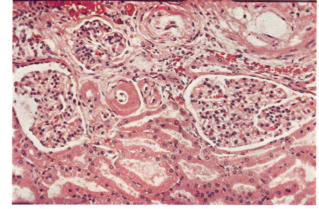

10.20 Hypertensive nephrosclerosis

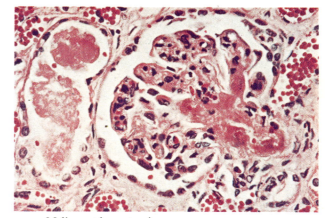

10.21 Malignant hypertension

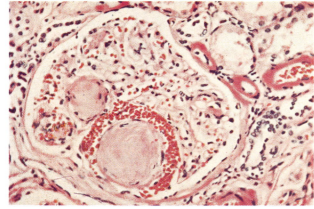

10.22 Diabetic glomerulosclerosis

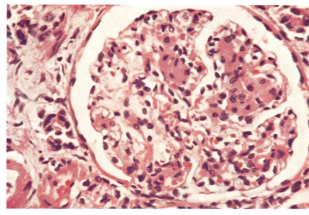

10.23 Diabetic glomerulosclerosis

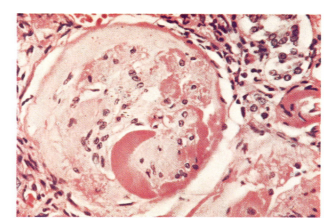

10.24 Diabetic glomerulosclerosis

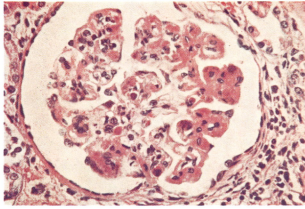

10.25 Systemic lupus erythematosus: kidney

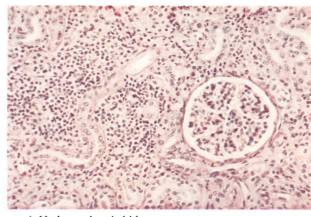

10.26 Hydronephrotic kidney

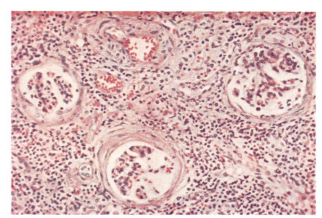

10.27 Hydronephrotic kidney

10.19–10.21 Hypertensive nephrosclerosis. 10.19 and **10.20** The patient had 'benign' hypertension. **10.19** In this arcuate artery, the muscle fibres of the hypertrophied media have been largely replaced by fibrous tissue. The internal elastic lamina is intact and appears to be augmented by wavy eosinophilic fibrils resembling elastic tissue (elastosis) in the intima. The intima shows the greatest changes of all. It is very thick, consisting of cellular connective tissue, so that the lumen of the vessels is greatly reduced. This may eventually lead to renal failure. **10.20** The smaller vessels are equally affected. The media of the small artery (top right) is fibrous, the intima is thickened and the lumen is very small. The arterioles (left of centre) show deposition of pink hyaline in the subintima and are severely stenosed (arteriolosclerosis). The smallest glomerulus has no tubules round it but the other glomeruli are nearer normal in size and appearance and have convoluted tubules (bottom) associated with them. Changes in the blood vessels as a result of hypertension lead to ischaemia and atrophy of the renal tissue, and if severe enough can eventually cause renal failure. They also add to the destructive effects of chronic pyelonephritis and chronic glomerulonephritis. **10.21** This patient suffered from 'malignant' hypertension. Histologically this syndrome is characterised by necrosis of the afferent arteriole and sometimes, as here, part of the adjacent glomerular tuft. The necrotic tissue (right of centre) is deeply eosinophilic (fibrinoid necrosis). The rest of the tuft is shrunken and slightly fibrosed. The epithelial cells lining Bowman's capsule are prominent. There is a dense protein cast in the tubule (left). The patient had congestive heart failure and the capillary bed is very congested. **10.22–10.24 Diabetic glomerulosclerosis. 10.22** This shows the classical Kimmelstiel-Wilson lesion. These are rounded acellular hyaline nodules in the glomerular tuft. The red cells surrounding the largest body are within a greatly dilated capillary. There is also a considerable deposit of hyaline material in the subintima of the arteriole (right) and in Bowman's capsule. **10.23** and **10.24** illustrate more diffuse forms of diabetic glomerulosclerosis. **10.23** There is patchy diffuse infiltration of the glomerular tuft with eosinophilic material which appears to have been deposited in the basement membrane. In places this has led to obliteration of the capillary bed. The afferent arteriole (bottom left) shows some hyaline change. **10.24** This is a much more advanced lesion than 10.22 and 10.23 and it is doubtful if any blood could flow through such a glomerulus. The infiltrate stains intensely red (exudative lesions) and is almost fibrinoid in appearance but the nuclei within it appear reasonably healthy. Diabetic glomerulosclerosis may eventually lead to a nephrotic syndrome and renal failure. Diabetic subjects are also liable to chronic pyelonephritis and papillary necrosis. **10.25 Systemic lupus erythematosus: kidney.** The glomerular tuft is excessively lobulated and the walls of some of the capillaries are infiltrated with a homogeneous material. This produces a 'wire-loop' appearance. Small dense rather basophilic 'thrombi' are present within some of the dilated capillaries and there may be focal proliferation of endothelial cells. Severe lesions may produce a nephrotic syndrome. **10.26** and **10.27 Hydronephrotic kidney. 10.26** Low power examination showed loss of many nephrons. This glomerular tuft appears relatively normal apart from slight fibrous thickening of Bowman's capsule. Some tubular atrophy is evident but the most marked feature is the intense lymphocytic infiltration of the interstitial tissue. **10.27** Characteristically the tubules are severely and disproportionately affected. Most of them have disappeared and the few that remain are atrophic and lack a lumen. The interstitial tissue is heavily infiltrated with lymphocytes. The glomeruli are small and excessively lobulated but their capillaries remain patent and there is no fibrosis. However Bowman's capsule is thick and fibrous.

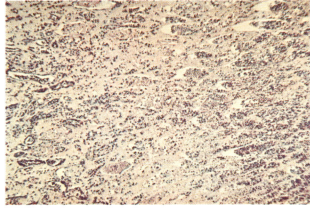

10.28 Necrosis: renal papilla

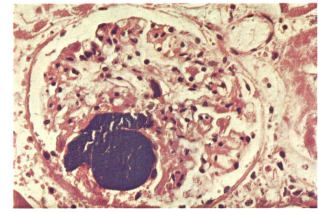

10.29 Focal embolic nephritis

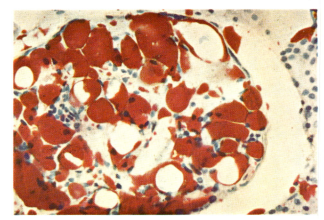

10.30 Fat embolism: kidney

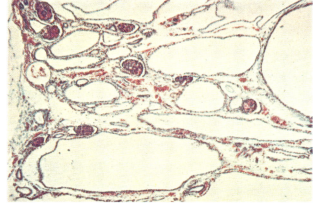

10.31 Congenital polycystic kidney

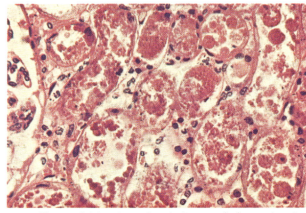

10.32 Haemoglobinuric nephrosis (acute tubular nephrosis; lower nephron nephrosis)

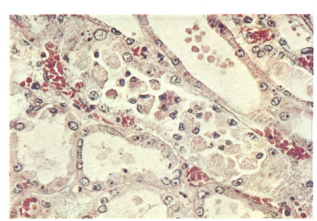

10.33 Acute tubular nephrosis (lower nephron nephrosis)

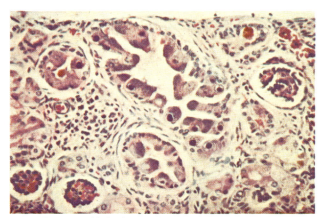

10.34 Cytomegalic inclusion disease: kidney

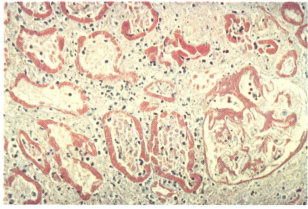

10.35 Recent infarct: kidney

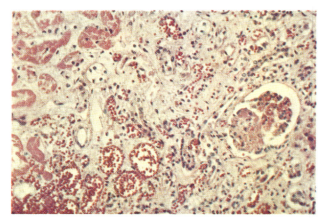

10.36 Recent infarct: kidney

10.28 Necrosis: renal papilla. The proximal part of the papilla (left) is viable but the tissue towards the tip is necrotic and disintegrating. The small spaces are collecting tubules full of bacteria and necrotic cellular debris. There is a remarkable lack of leucocytic response at the junction (left of centre) of the living and necrotic tissues. Papillary necrosis is a complication of acute pyelonephritis and is usually associated with diabetes mellitus or, less commonly, with urinary obstruction. Sometimes it is associated with abuse of analgesic drugs. **10.29 Focal embolic nephritis.** One large clump and one small clump of bacteria (stained deep blue) occupy part of the glomerular tuft. There is a little necrosis around them but no inflammatory reaction. The patient had subacute bacterial endocarditis and the organisms (S. viridans) reached the glomerulus in a small embolus from an infected vegetation on the cusp of the mitral valve. This is an uncommon variety of the focal glomerulonephritis in subacute bacterial endocarditis. More often bacteria are not seen and the focal inflammatory foci in the glomeruli probably have an allergic basis. **10.30 Fat embolism: kidney.** This is a frozen section of kidney from a young woman who died from multiple injuries which included a fractured femur. The glomerular capillaries are distended with fat globules and a very small amount of fat is present in the subcapsular space (right). The gaps in some droplets are caused by fat dissolving in the stain (Sudan IV). Death from fat embolism is often attributable to lesions in the central nervous system. **10.31 Congenital polycystic kidney.** The capsule of the kidney is on the left. Large numbers of cysts lined by flattened epithelium are present. The remaining glomeruli look fairly healthy but there are no normal secretory tubules. **10.32 Haemoglobinuric nephrosis (acute tubular nephrosis; lower nephron nephrosis).** The lesion is essentially tubular and the glomerulus, part of which is visible on the left, showed no abnormality. The tubules (convoluted tubules and loop of Henle) contain eosinophilic debris which appears to block the lumen of most of

them. Some of the material is haemoglobin and some consists of necrotic tubular epithelium. As a result of the destruction of tubular epithelium many of the tubules have no cellular lining. The others are lined by very flat, probably regenerating, cells. This patient died from Blackwater fever, in which haemoglobinuria follows massive intravascular haemolysis. **10.33 Acute tubular nephrosis (lower nephron nephrosis).** Most of the tubular epithelium has died and sloughed off into the lumen of the convoluted tubules. There have been considerable attempts at repair by the surviving cells and already the tubules are lined by flat greatly elongated cells. Despite this the patient died from renal failure seven days after an operation for relief of constrictive pericarditis. The kidney is very hyperaemic. **10.34 Cytomegalic inclusion disease: kidney.** The tubular epithelial cells are greatly swollen and large inclusions are present within the nuclei. This disease is an infection of infants with the salivary gland virus and similar inclusions were present in the salivary glands. It also occurs in older subjects in whom the immune response is deficient, as in Hodgkin's disease or because of therapy. **10.35** and **10.36 Recent infarct: kidney. 10.35** The lesion is a few days old and the tissue, consisting of a glomerulus (right) and its associated tubules, is completely necrotic. The nuclei have either completely dissolved (karyolysis) or broken down into deep blue fragments. Note also the opaque deep pink appearance of the necrotic cytoplasm of the tubular epithelium. **10.36** This is the edge of the lesion. The cells lining the tubules (left) are necrotic; there is no nuclear staining and the cytoplasm is deeply eosinophilic. The tissues in the right half of the picture are probably viable though one half of the glomerulus appears necrotic. The capillaries of the boundary zone are greatly distended and from them many cells would shortly have emigrated to digest the dead tissue. The stroma is oedematous with separation of the tubules.

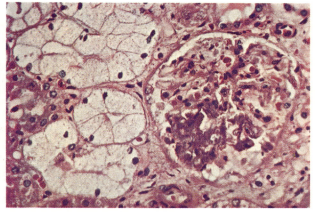

10.37 Metastatic calcification: kidney

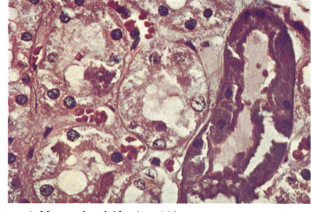

10.38 Metastatic calcification: kidney

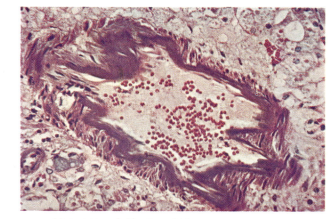

10.39 Metastatic calcification: kidney

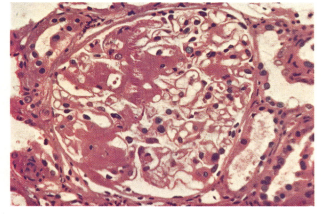

10.40 Amyloid disease: kidney

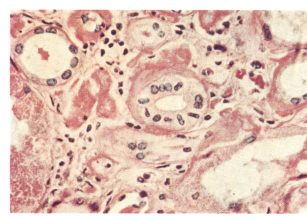

10.41 Amyloid disease: kidney

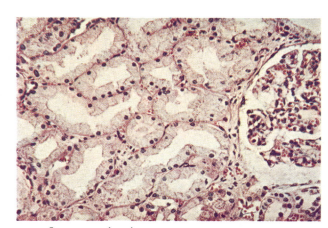

10.42 Sucrose nephrosis

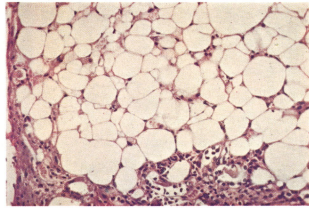

10.43 Lipoma: kidney

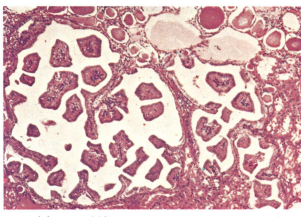

10.44 Adenoma: kidney

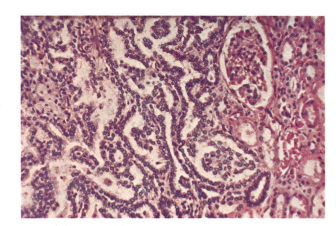

10.45 Adenoma: kidney

10.37–10.39 Metastatic calcification: kidney. The patient had a carcinoma of the parathyroid gland and died from hyperparathyroidism and renal failure. **10.37** Parts of the glomerular tuft are calcified and stain deep blue. The cells of the convoluted tubules are extremely hydropic, a change usually associated with intravenous administration of hypertonic sucrose solution and potassium deficiency. **10.38** Many of the epithelial cells of the convoluted tubules have calcified, some completely (right). In others the cytoplasmic lesion is still focal (centre left). There is also early deposition of calcium in the basement membranes of the tubules. Nuclei are still present within the completely calcified cells but they are small and pyknotic and presumably the cells are dead. They appear to be firmly adherent to the cast in the lumen. Calcified cells often slough off and form calcium casts. **10.39** Elastic tissue is particularly apt to calcify and the internal elastic lamina of this artery is calcified and deeply basophilic. The muscle coats are only slightly affected. Vascular calcification is severe in secondary (renal) hyperparathyroidism in which the blood phosphate level is increased. **10.40** and **10.41 Amyloid disease: kidney.** The lesion was secondary to chronic pulmonary tuberculosis. **10.40** The glomerular tuft is large but the basement membrane of the capillaries is infiltrated to a varying degree by pink acellular amyloid. The lumen of the more severely affected vessels is probably obliterated. The tubules are still relatively unaffected. Severe lesions render the glomeruli functionless. **10.41** The hyaline amyloid material has also infiltrated the basement membrane of the collecting tubules and the loop of Henle (centre). The convoluted tubule (bottom left) is free from deposit but its epithelial cells are swollen and granular as a result of the proteinuria produced by the disease. **10.42 Sucrose nephrosis.** This tubular lesion was caused by the intravenous administration of concentrated sucrose. The epithelial cells lining the convoluted tubules are greatly swollen from cytoplasmic oedema (hydropic degeneration). The glomerulus is unaffected. **10.43 Lipoma: kidney.** Lipomas are generally found in the renal cortex and this example is located beneath the renal capsule (left). It consists of mature fat cells and there is no fibrous capsule separating it from the renal tissue (bottom). Sometimes smooth muscle, cartilage or connective tissue are present along with the fat; and lesions of this type are found in most cases of tuberous sclerosis. Intrarenal lipomas should not be confused with the fatty replacement of renal tissue destroyed by inflammatory processes. **10.44** and **10.45 Adenoma: kidney. 10.44** Typically the tumour is a papillary cystadenoma. The stroma of the epithelium-covered papillary processes is infiltrated with lymphocytes. There is no fibrous capsule and the tumour merges with the surrounding renal tissue. The tubules (top) contain dense 'colloid' casts and both kidneys were severely affected by chronic pyelonephritis. **10.45** This tumour consists of dark-staining cuboidal epithelial cells which form a complex series of tubules. The nuclei of these cells are regular in size and shape and exhibit no mitotic activity and the stroma of mature connective tissue is not unduly vascular. The 'capsule' of the tumour is compressed renal tissue (right).

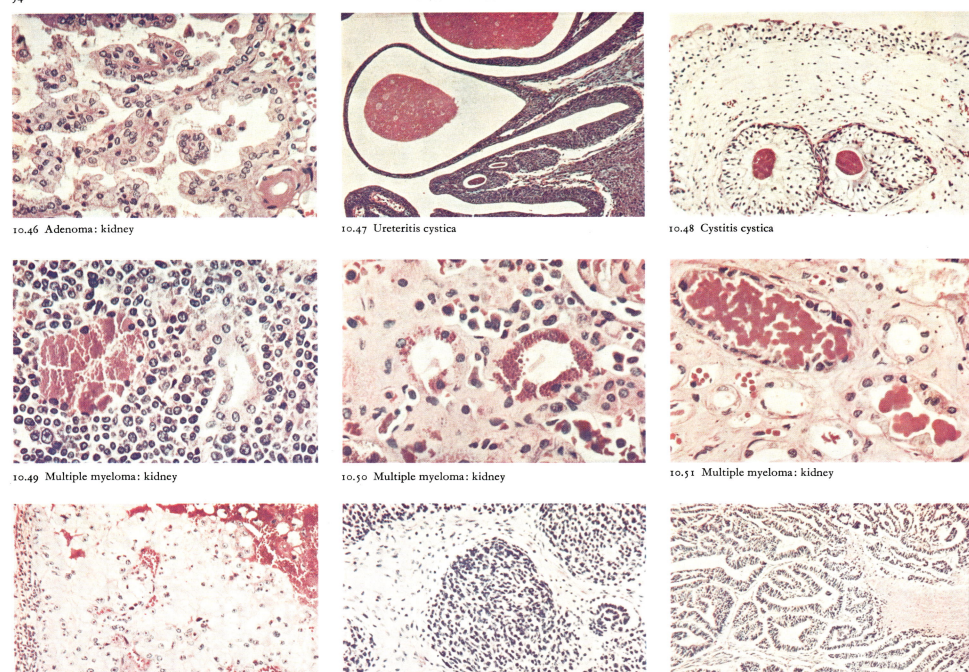

10.46 Adenoma: kidney

10.47 Ureteritis cystica

10.48 Cystitis cystica

10.49 Multiple myeloma: kidney

10.50 Multiple myeloma: kidney

10.51 Multiple myeloma: kidney

10.52 Primary adenocarcinoma: kidney

10.53 Nephroblastoma (Wilms' tumour): kidney

10.54 Nephroblastoma: kidney

10.46 Adenoma: kidney. The tumour bears some resemblance to a renal carcinoma but the epithelial cells covering the finger-like processes are well-differentiated and although there is mitotic activity pleomorphism is slight. There is no fibrous capsule and the tumour is bounded only by renal tissue (right). Tumours less than 3 cm. diameter can be safely called adenomas however, since they almost never metastasize. The arteriole (bottom right) is severely sclerotic. **10.47 Ureteritis cystica.** The transitional epithelium lining the ureter has grown into the tunica propria to form the cell-nests of von Brunn. Pink fluid has collected in the centre of the nests and two of them have become cystic. The epithelium lining the cysts has flattened. Ureteritis cystica is often associated with pyelitis and there is some lymphocytic infiltration of the lamina propria. **10.48 Cystitis cystica.** The bladder is affected in this case. The two cell nests show very early cyst formation and each contains a small amount of dense secretion. The transitional epithelial cells lining the bladder are swollen and oedematous, with clear, unstained cytoplasm and the epithelium of the cell nests has a similar appearance. The vascular connective tissue of the tunica propria is also extremely oedematous but only scanty lymphocytes and plasma cells are present. **10.49–10.51 Multiple myeloma: kidney. 10.49** The interstitial tissue of the kidney is packed with plasma cells of widely varying degrees of maturity. The nuclear irregularity and the prominent nucleoli (bottom left) in some of the plasma cells also suggest that the infiltrate is neoplastic and not inflammatory. The cells lining the convoluted tubule (left) are laden with dense protein droplets, the result of proteinuria. **10.50** This demonstrates even more clearly the large deeply eosinophilic protein droplets in the cytoplasm of the epithelial cells lining the convoluted tubules. These droplets are probably formed by reabsorption of protein from the secretion in the lumen of the tubules. Plasma cells are scattered throughout the interstitial tissue. **10.51** Deeply eosinophilic material, presumably precipitated protein, fills the lumen of two collecting tubules. This material forms very dense-looking casts, which seem to be pressing on and causing atrophy and even destruction of the epithelial cells. These casts block the tubules and sometimes provoke a granulomatous foreign-body reaction and giant cell formation with degeneration of the affected nephron. **10.52 Primary adenocarcinoma: kidney.** This is the so-called hypernephroma of kidney. It consists of sheets of large cells which possess abundant pale foamy (lipid-rich) cytoplasm. The lipid within the cells gives the tumour a characteristic yellow colour. The nucleoli are prominent but no mitotic figures are evident. The scanty stroma consists largely of thin-walled vessels which tend to rupture giving rise to haemorrhage (top right), though one part is more fibrous and heavily infiltrated with lymphocytes (left). A papillary or tubular structure is sometimes present and a small tumour may be mistaken for an adenoma. Renal carcinoma tends to metastasize by the blood stream to bones or lung. **10.53** and **10.54 Nephroblastoma (Wilms' tumour): kidney.** This rare mixed tumour is derived from primitive mesodermal cells. **10.53** A mixture of 'epithelial' and connective tissue elements is present in this lesion. The epithelial cells have large basophilic nuclei and very little cytoplasm. These cells mostly form masses of undifferentiated tissue but a small glomerulus-like structure (right) is evident. The epithelial cells also sometimes form tubules. The connective tissue element is myxomatous but occasionally it is sarcomatous and other tissues such as muscle or cartilage are present. **10.54** The epithelial element in this part of the tumour forms large, irregular tubules. There is a considerable amount of necrosis (centre right).

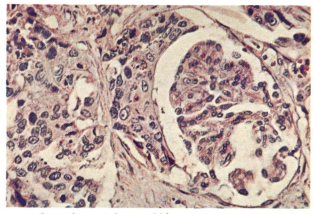

10.55 Secondary carcinoma: kidney

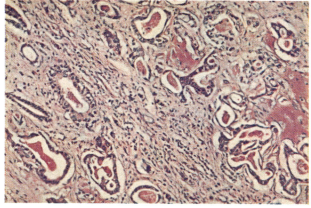

10.56 Primary adenocarcinoma: renal pelvis

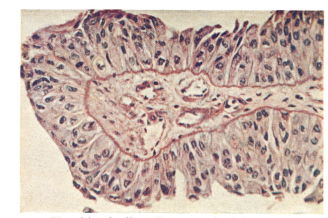

10.57 Transitional cell papilloma: renal pelvis

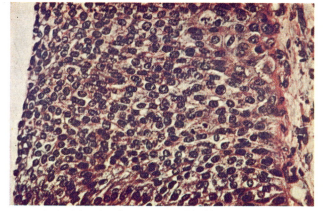

10.58 Transitional cell carcinoma: bladder

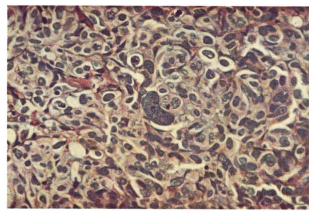

10.59 Transitional cell carcinoma: bladder

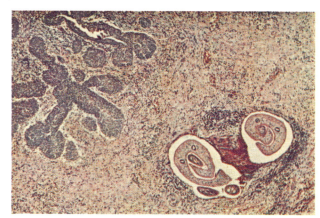

10.60 Schistosomiasis (Bilharziasis): bladder

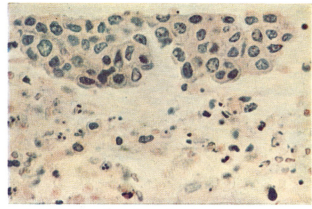

10.61 Malignant cells: urinary deposit

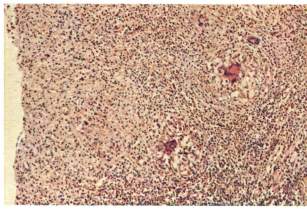

10.62 Tuberculosis: ureter

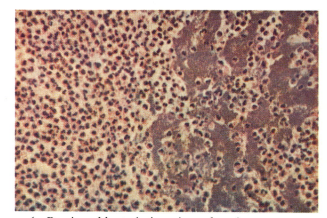

10.63 Pyuria and bacteriuria: urinary deposit

10.55 Secondary carcinoma: kidney. The primary was an undifferentiated carcinoma of bronchus. Part of the main secondary deposit is visible on the left. From it cells have invaded the subcapsular space to form a 'crescent'. The tumour cells are large and exhibit considerable nuclear pleomorphism. A few cells in the main deposit are necrotic and their nuclei are fragmenting. **10.56 Primary adenocarcinoma: renal pelvis.** This is a rare tumour which probably arises from the epithelium of the distal collecting tubules or by metaplasia of renal pelvic epithelium. The cells form irregular large acini which contain eosinophilic material. They are surrounded by abundant fibrous stroma. The appearances are similar to the better-known adenocarcinoma of bladder. **10.57 Transitional cell papilloma: renal pelvis.** Because of their tendency to recur, tumours of this type should be regarded as well-differentiated papillary carcinomas. The vascular core of connective tissue is covered with transitional epithelial cells that show some loss of polarity. There is also fairly marked nuclear pleomorphism and a mitotic figure is evident. The basement membrane is intact. **10.58 and 10.59 Transitional cell carcinoma: bladder. 10.58** Clinically this was a sessile shaggy polyp. The epithelial cell layer is very thick and basophilic, the nucleus/cytoplasm ratio being high. However the cells rest upon an intact basement membrane. The stroma (right) consists of loose areolar tissue. **10.59** This is a much more malignant tumour than 10.58. This field is deep in the muscle coats of the bladder and it shows invasion by cells which though they still resemble transitional epithelium show great nuclear pleomorphism and basophilia. One nucleus (centre) is relatively enormous. The nucleoli are

prominent. There are no mitotic figures here but they were fairly numerous elsewhere in the tumour. The stroma is scanty. **10.60 Schistosomiasis (Bilharziasis): bladder.** The parasite is S. haematobium. A gravid adult female worm (lower right), containing several ova, lies in the submucosal connective tissues of the bladder wall. There is an intense cellular infiltrate around the worm, many of the cells being eosinophil leucocytes, and a considerable fibrosis has occurred. The overlying transitional epithelium (top left) shows intense hyperplasia, with downgrowths of finger-like processes. This hyperplasia sometimes proceeds to malignancy. **10.61 Malignant cells: urinary deposit.** This is a smear of the urinary deposit from a patient with a transitional carcinoma of bladder and it shows a clump of malignant epithelial cells. The large size and pleomorphism of the tumour cell nuclei and the prominence of the nucleoli are evidence of the neoplastic nature of the cells. There are also a few individual malignant cells, as well as red cells and polymorphs. **10.62 Tuberculosis: ureter.** The transitional epithelium has disappeared and the ureter is lined with tuberculous granulation tissue. This is intensely cellular, the cells being epithelioid cells and lymphocytes. There are several follicles and in two of these a multinucleated giant cell is present. Fibrous tissue formation is beginning, particularly around the follicles. **10.63 Pyuria and bacteriuria.** This is a section of the urinary sediment from a case of suspected bladder neoplasm. Large numbers of polymorphs and bacteria are present but there are no malignant cells.

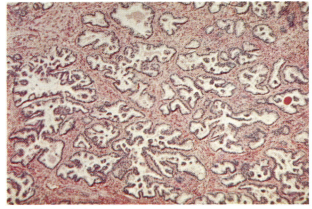

11.1 Hyperplasia: prostate

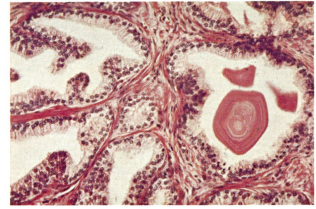

11.2 Hyperplasia: prostate

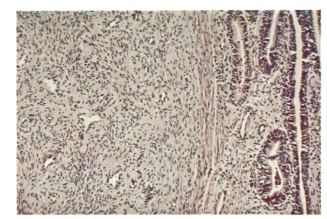

11.3 Hyperplasia: prostate

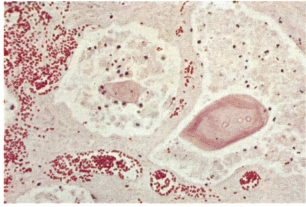

11.4 Infarct: prostate

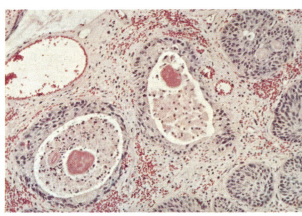

11.5 Infarct and squamous metaplasia: prostate

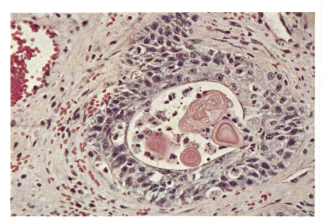

11.6 Infarct and squamous metaplasia: prostate

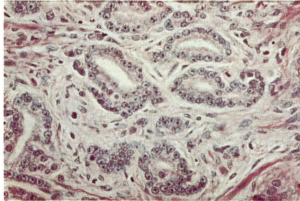

11.7 Primary adenocarcinoma: prostate

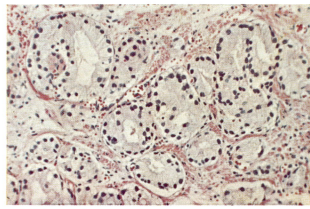

11.8 Primary adenocarcinoma: prostate

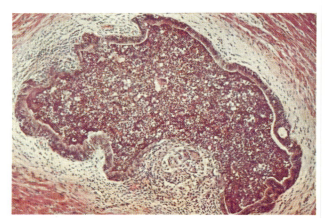

11.9 Tuberculosis: epididymis

11.1–11.3 Hyperplasia: prostate. 11.1 This is a section of one of the many nodules in the enlarged organ. It consists of glands and fibromuscular stroma. The glands are tortuous and intraluminal growth of epithelium has occurred. A few glands contain secretion and in one there is a corpus amylaceum (right of centre). **11.2** The cells lining the glands are uniformly tall fully-differentiated columnar cells, with a marked tendency to intra-acinar proliferation. The stroma is a mixture of smooth muscle and fibrous (paler-staining) connective tissue. Lamination is marked in the corpus amylaceum (right). **11.3** In this case the nodule consists entirely of fibromuscular tissue and glandular elements are lacking. There is a 'capsule' which consists largely of compressed smooth muscle. Some believe that fibromuscular hyperplasia precedes glandular hyperplasia. The epithelial structures on the right are periurethral ducts. **11.4 Infarct: prostate.** The prostatic tissue is necrotic and the epithelium lining the acini has disappeared. The acini contain remnants of necrotic cells and corpora amylacea. The capillaries are very dilated and there is considerable haemorrhage. **11.5** and **11.6 Infarct and squamous metaplasia: prostate. 11.5** This is the edge of the lesion shown in 11.4. The prostatic epithelium is hyperplastic. It either fills the acini or forms a thick lining layer and squamous metaplasia is evident (right). There is haemorrhage into the stroma of the gland and necrotic cell debris and corpora amylacea are present within the acini. **11.6** This shows in detail the squamous metaplasia of the epithelial cells. The cells also show a certain amount of pleomorphism but this form of epithelial

overgrowth should not be mistaken for carcinoma. Squamous carcinoma is a rare tumour of prostate whereas squamous metaplasia is not an uncommon finding and may be induced by oestrogen therapy. The lumen contains corpora amylacea and fragments of dead cells. There is haemorrhage into the necrotic stroma. **11.7** and **11.8 Primary adenocarcinoma: prostate. 11.7** The epithelial cells are of uniform size and shape but have relatively large nuclei and the prominence of the nucleoli is particularly striking. The acini are small and irregular in shape and the architecture is clearly abnormal. The stroma consists of fibrous tissue and smooth muscle fibres. The regularity of cells, nuclei and acini occasionally cause difficulty in differentiating carcinoma from hyperplasia, and in these circumstances capsular or lymphatic invasion must be carefully searched for. Abnormality of general architecture should also be sought. **11.8** The malignant cells of the adenocarcinoma are tall columnar mucin-secreting cells which have deeply basophilic nuclei that are not markedly pleomorphic. However the acini are very closely packed and stroma is lacking between them: features which suggest malignancy. There is considerable haemorrhage into the stroma, perhaps the result of operation trauma. **11.9 Tuberculosis: epididymis.** A duct is full of tuberculous pus which consists of cellular debris that is largely necrotic. The cells include polymorphs and multinucleate giant cells. A small follicle is present in the wall of the duct (bottom centre) and the epithelium over it has ulcerated. The tissue round the duct consists of smooth muscle and fibrous tissue heavily infiltrated with chronic inflammatory cells.

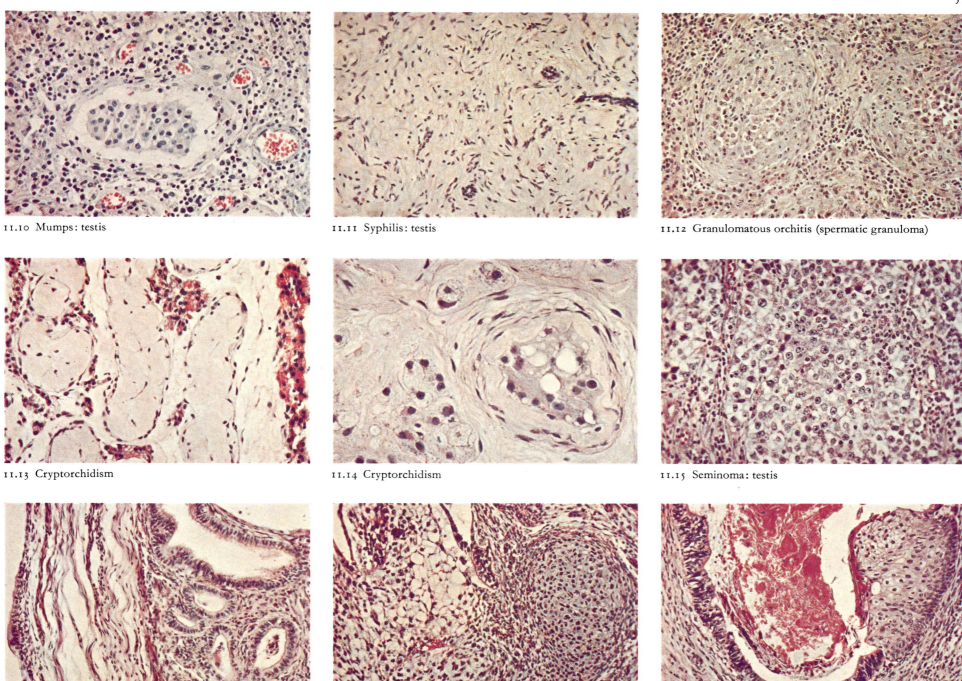

11.10 Mumps: testis

11.11 Syphilis: testis

11.12 Granulomatous orchitis (spermatic granuloma)

11.13 Cryptorchidism

11.14 Cryptorchidism

11.15 Seminoma: testis

11.16 Differentiated teratoma: testis

11.17 Malignant teratoma: testis

11.18 Differentiated teratoma: testis

11.10 Mumps: testis. The organ is very severely affected and this shows one of the few recognisable seminiferous tubules that remained. There is no spermatogenesis and the cells in the lumen are Sertoli cells. The surrounding tissues are necrotic and heavily infiltrated with lymphocytes and plasma cells. **11.11 Syphilis: testis.** The testis was small and hard. There is diffuse interstitial fibrosis, with complete loss of seminiferous tubules and interstitial cells. A few small ductules survive. Syphilitic orchitis may also take the form of one or more gummas. **11.12 Granulomatous orchitis (spermatic granuloma).** In this condition the contents of the seminiferous tubules are released into the interstitial tissues and produce a tuberculoid granulomatous reaction there. The normal tissues have been replaced by epithelioid cells and plasma cells, the epithelioid cells forming two follicles which are enclosed in fibrous tissue. A few cells in the centre are degenerate and probably necrotic. No spermatozoa are visible here but they are sometimes numerous. **11.13 and 11.14 Cryptorchidism. 11.13** The tubules of this undescended testis are completely hyalinised but interstitial (Leydig) cells are present in large numbers. The number of these cells varies considerably in cryptorchidism and sometimes the testis consists almost entirely of fibrous tissue. **11.14** In this testis too, spermatogenesis is lacking but Sertoli cells fill the lumen of the spermatic tubules. The basement membrane of the tubule is very thick and fibrous. There are many interstitial cells (left) but their granular cytoplasm is unusually pale-staining. **11.15 Seminoma: testis.** This neoplasm arises from the germinal (seminiferous) epi-

thelium of the mature or maturing testis. The tumour cells are large, polyhedral and closely packed. They are very uniform and have abundant clear or foamy cytoplasm. The nucleoli are very prominent and in some nuclei they are multiple. An occasional nucleus is pyknotic. The delicate fibrous stroma is heavily infiltrated with lymphocytes. **11.16–11.18 Teratoma: testis.** The teratoma contains many tissue structures foreign to the normal testis. These tissues vary in their degree of differentiation and sometimes adopt an 'organoid' arrangement. **11.16 Differentiated teratoma.** This is a differentiated teratoma, consisting of mature tissues. The lumen of a large cyst is visible on the left, lined by flattened epithelium. The epithelium lining the small ducts and cysts (right) is tall columnar. The stroma is densely fibrous. The mixture of cystic glands and fibrous tissue accounts for the old name of fibrocystic disease of testis. **11.17 Malignant teratoma.** Here the tissues are more primitive and embryonic and consist of cartilage (right) and myxomatous connective tissue (left). There are also epithelium-lined spaces (top left). **11.18 Differentiated teratoma.** In differentiated teratomas squamous epithelium is often abundant and this shows a fibrous-walled cyst full of keratinous squames derived from the lining of stratified squamous epithelium (right). Part of the cyst is lined by columnar epithelium (below and left). The surrounding fibrous tissue is infiltrated by lymphocytes. It should not be assumed that a differentiated teratoma of testis will inevitably behave like a benign neoplasm, since malignant areas are readily overlooked during histological examination.

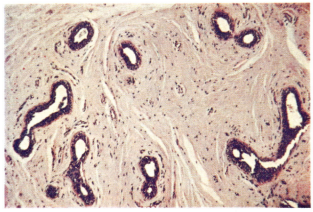

12.1 Mammary dysplasia (cystic hyperplasia; chronic mastitis)

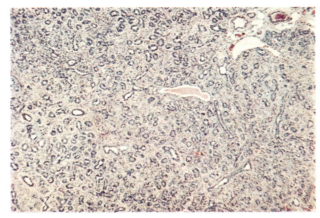

12.2 Mammary dysplasia

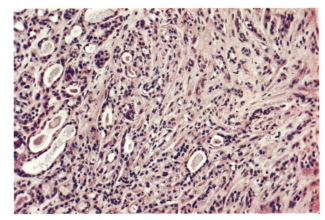

12.3 Mammary dysplasia

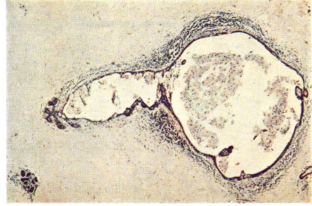

12.4 Mammary dysplasia

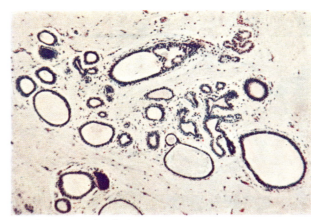

12.5 Mammary dysplasia

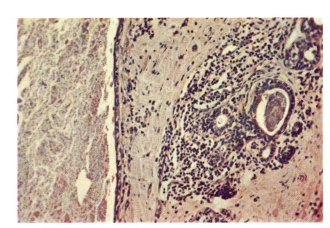

12.6 Mammary dysplasia

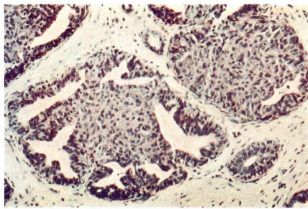

12.7 Mammary dysplasia

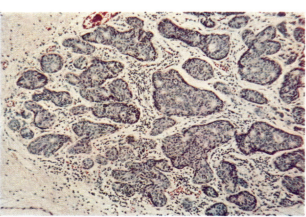

12.8 Intraduct carcinoma: breast

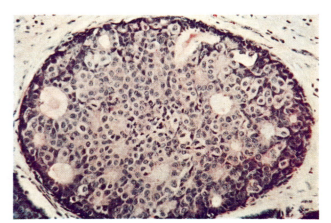

12.9 Intraduct carcinoma: breast

12.1–12.7 Mammary dysplasia (cystic hyperplasia; chronic mastitis). 12.1 The epithelial structures of the lobule show no abnormality but the lobular connective tissue is much more fibrous than normal. This is mazoplasia. **12.2** and **12.3** The epithelium has proliferated greatly to form many new ductules and groups of cells which are embedded in dense fibrous stroma. This is sclerosing adenosis. In 12.3 the appearances suggest malignancy but the cells are fairly regular in form. Usually a lobular pattern is visible on low power examination and helps to distinguish this condition from carcinoma. **12.4** This shows a duct that has undergone cystic dilatation. This lumen is full of amorphous and cellular debris and there is infiltration of the surrounding tissues by chronic inflammatory cells. **12.5** Many of the ductules are dilated and cystic, and the stroma of the lobules is much more fibrous than normal. There is also moderate lymphocytic infiltration. **12.6** This is part of the wall of a large cyst. The lumen (left) is full of amor- phous debris and the lining epithelium is very flat and atrophic and the stroma in the vicinity is densely fibrous. There is intense lymphocytic infiltration around the neighbouring ducts (right). **12.7** The epithelial cells have proliferated almost to fill the lumen of two ducts. However the cells are fairly regular in form and mitotic activity is not evident. This is epitheliosis. It is some- times difficult to distinguish epitheliosis from intraduct carcinoma and it may be that mammary dysplasia predisposes to the development of carcinoma. **12.8** and **12.9 Intraduct carcinoma: breast. 12.8** Each of the ductules in this lobule is distended with proliferated epithelial cells. The stroma of the lobule is overrun with lymphocytes. **12.9** High power examination of one of the ductules in 12.8 shows that the epithelial cells are malignant. They are large, the nucleus/ cytoplasm ratio is relatively high, and there are mitotic figures. The cells are also forming imperfect acini and producing a cribriform pattern. A few of the cells in the centre are necrotic.

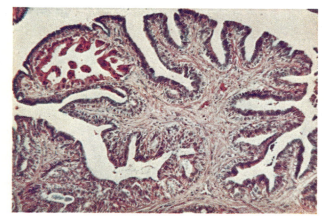

12.10 Papilloma: breast

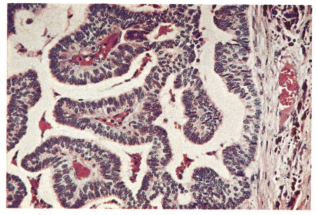

12.11 Primary papilliferous adenocarcinoma: breast

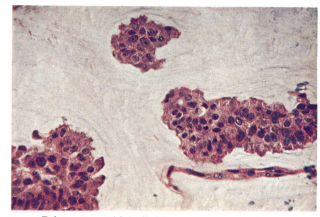

12.12 Primary mucoid (colloid) carcinoma: breast

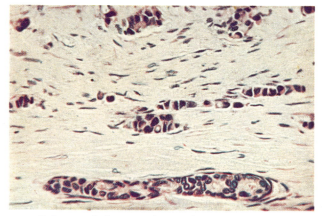

12.13 Primary scirrhous carcinoma: breast

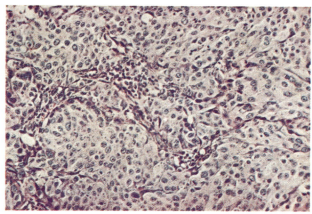

12.14 Primary medullary carcinoma: breast

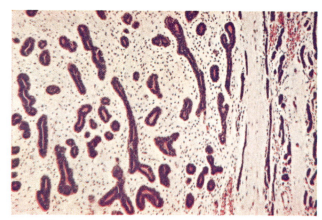

12.15 Fibroadenoma: breast

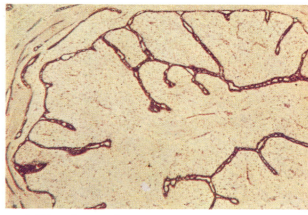

12.16 Fibroadenoma: breast

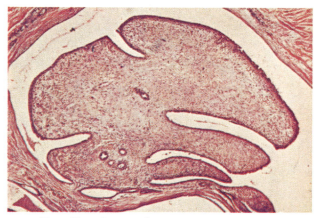

12.17 Giant fibroadenoma: breast

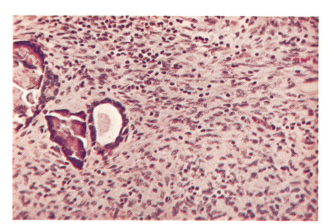

12.18 Primary sarcoma: breast

12.10 Papilloma: breast. The lesion was a polypoid mass (1.5 cm. diameter) distending a main duct just beneath the nipple. It has a well-developed densely fibrous stroma and the covering epithelium is hyperplastic. However, on close examination the cells showed no undue proliferative activity, and the lesion is benign. There is apocrine metaplasia of the epithelium in one part (top left). **12.11 Primary papilliferous adenocarcinoma: breast.** The tumour cells form cystic spaces into which numerous papilliform processes project. These have a vascular fibrous stroma and are covered by columnar epithelial cells several layers thick. Haemorrhage has occurred at the edge of the tumour (right) and haemosiderin-laden macrophages are present. **12.12 Primary mucoid (colloid) carcinoma: breast.** Compact clusters of malignant cells float in mucin. The mucin is epithelial in origin, secreted by the neoplastic cells. A stromal blood vessel is visible (bottom right). **12.13 Primary scirrhous carcinoma: breast.** The tumour cells lie in cords and small clumps in a very dense fibrous tissue stroma. The nuclei of the tumour cells are very irregular and basophilic. There is an attempt at acinus formation (bottom right). Despite the abundance and density of the stroma, scirrhous carcinomas metastasize readily. They are the commonest variety of breast carcinoma. **12.14 Primary medullary carcinoma: breast.** The tumour was a round soft (encephaloid) mass 7 cm. in diameter. The malignant epithelial cells are large, close-packed and polyhedral, with weakly basophilic cytoplasm. The nucleoli are prominent. They form large groups or sheets, separated by a scanty connective tissue stroma. The stroma of these tumours is often heavily infiltrated with lymphocytes. **12.15** and **12.16**

Fibroadenoma: breast. 12.15 The pattern is pericanalicular, the lesion consisting of ductules and glands embedded in a loose connective tissue stroma. There is a well-formed fibrous capsule and the adjacent breast tissue (right) is compressed. **12.16** The pattern is intracanalicular. Stromal overgrowth predominates and the lesion thus consists of a lobulated mass of myxoid connective tissue, the surface of each lobule being covered by epithelium. The capsule (top and left) is fibrous and the adjacent breast elements are compressed. Most fibroadenomas are a mixture of pericanalicular and intracanalicular structures. **12.17 Giant fibroadenoma: breast.** This is only a small part of the tumour which was 10 cm. diameter. A large polypoid mass of connective tissue, covered by a thick layer of hyperplastic epithelium, projects into a cystic ductule which is lined by very flat epithelial cells. Higher-power examination of the connective tissue reveals fairly numerous mitotic figures, and a tumour like this should be treated as a sarcoma of low-grade malignancy. **12.18 Primary sarcoma: breast.** This lesion developed in a fibroadenoma that had been present for some years and which started to grow after the menopause. It is a spindle cell sarcoma. The cell boundaries are not well-defined and there is a considerable amount of fibrillary intercellular substance. Many lymphocytes are present. The two ducts (left) may be breast structures 'caught up' in the tumour, though sometimes epithelial structures seem to form an actively-growing component of the tumour, and the tumour is virtually an adenosarcoma. Calcium deposition has occurred in the material in the lumen of one duct and in part of the tumour.

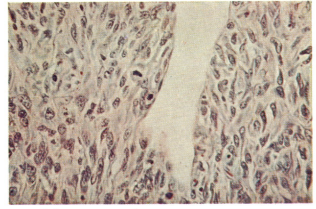

12.19 Primary sarcoma: breast

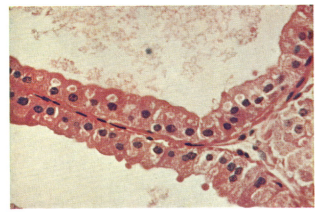

12.20 Apocrine metaplasia: breast

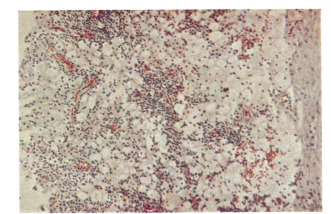

12.21 Fat necrosis: breast

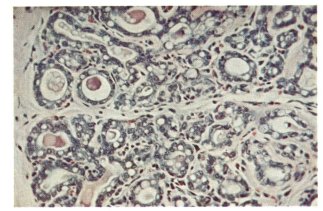

12.22 Pregnancy: breast

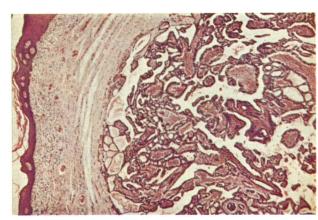

12.23 Hidradenoma: vulva

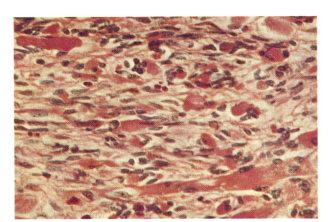

12.24 Mesodermal mixed tumour (botryoid sarcoma): vagina

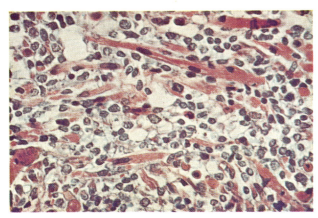

12.25 Mesodermal mixed tumour: vagina

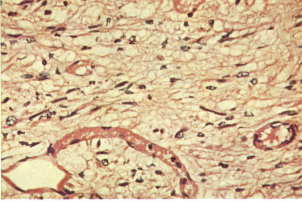

12.26 Mesodermal mixed tumour: bladder

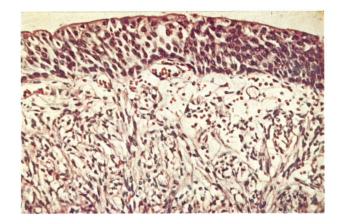

12.27 Mesodermal mixed tumour: bladder

12.19 Primary sarcoma: breast. This is a spindle-cell sarcoma. There is evidence of active growth in the form of mitotic activity and the cells have formed a certain amount of collagenous tissue. The space in the centre is an empty blood vessel. It has no proper wall and seems to be lined at least in part by tumour cells. **12.20 Apocrine metaplasia: breast.** Parts of two dilated, cystic ductules are seen. The cells lining them have abundant pink cytoplasm and closely resemble apocrine epithelium. Several cells demonstrate clearly the apocrine type of secretion in which the tip of the secreting cell buds off into the lumen. Apocrine metaplasia is most commonly seen in mammary dysplasia (cystic hyperplasia; chronic mastitis). **12.21 Fat necrosis: breast.** The lesion was a fixed hard lump, indistinguishable clinically from carcinoma. The necrotic fat has been phagocytosed by macrophages and invaded by capillaries. Organisation in this way has produced a cystic lesion enclosed in dense fibrous tissue (right) and lined by a vascular and cellular granulation tissue. Most of the cells in the granulation tissue are large foamy (lipid-laden) macrophages, though focal collections of lymphocytes and plasma cells are also present. The centre of the cyst (left) was filled with turbid fluid. **12.22 Pregnancy: breast.** The lobule has enlarged greatly, as a result of proliferation of the glandular epithelium. There are many new acini, embedded in a delicate stroma. The cuboidal epithelial cells contain secretory vacu-

oles and in a few acini (left) there is a little secretion. **12.23 Hidradenoma: vulva.** The surface of the skin is on the left. The lesion is a benign well-demarcated papilliferous growth, resembling an intraduct papilloma of breast. It has a well-formed fibrous stroma and is enclosed in a 'capsule' formed by compression of the surrounding connective tissues. Hidradenomas arise from epithelium of the apocrine sweat gland type. **12.24–12.27 Mesodermal mixed tumour (botryoid sarcoma).** This tumour arises from the urogenital mesenchyme and so may contain a wide variety of tissue elements. **12.24 and 12.25** In the female the lesion may arise in the mucosal stroma of the endometrium, cervix or vagina, and this example was in the vagina of a girl of 6 years. **12.24** Here it is rhabdomyosarcomatous, consisting of elongated cells which are differentiating to form striated muscle (bottom right). **12.25** In this part the cells are forming myofibrils which are not striated and structurally are much more like smooth muscle. **12.26 and 12.27** This neoplasm was in the bladder of a six year old boy. **12.26** It is myxosarcomatous, the vacuolated spaces containing the abundant mucinous ground-substance that gave the tumour its characteristic soft consistence. The pink-stained vessel is a capillary. **12.27** The striking feature is the virtually normal appearance of the bladder epithelium even though the underlying tissues have been completely replaced by the mucoid sarcomatous tissue.

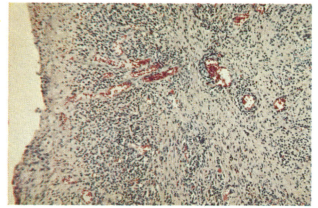

12.28 Chronic cervicitis

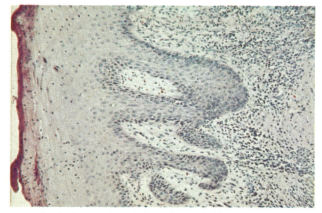

12.29 Leukokeratosis and chronic cervicitis

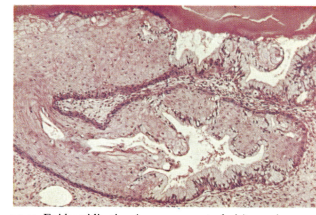

12.30 Epidermidization (squamous metaplasia): cervix

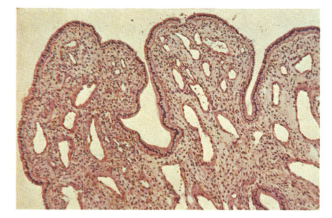

12.31 Endocervical polyp

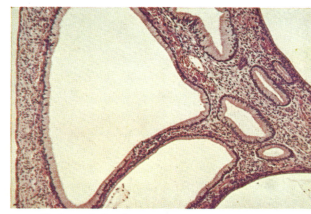

12.32 Endocervical polyp

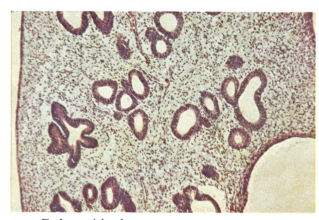

12.33 Endometrial polyp

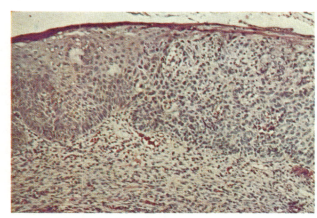

12.34 Carcinoma in situ: cervix

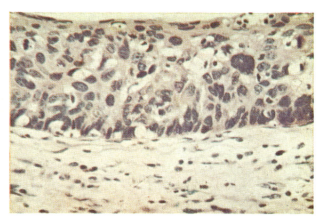

12.35 Carcinoma in situ: cervix

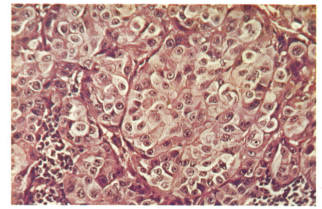

12.36 Primary squamous carcinoma: cervix

12.28 Chronic cervicitis. The epithelium (left) is ulcerated and the underlying tissues are hyperaemic and intensely infiltrated with lymphocytes and plasma cells. The ulcer is probably traumatic, from a pessary, and not to be confused with a cervical erosion. **12.29 Leukokeratosis and chronic cervicitis.** The clear glycogen-containing squamous epithelial cells of the normal cervix have been replaced by a non-glycogen-containing epithelium (left) which shows a considerable degree of hyperplasia. The surface layers are keratinised and there is epithelial downgrowth. Mitotic figures are present in the elongated epithelial processes. The underlying tissues (right) are heavily infiltrated with chronic inflammatory cells (lymphocytes and plasma cells). **12.30 Epidermidization (squamous metaplasia): cervix.** This is the external os, at the junction of the mucin-secreting columnar epithelium (right) that lines the cervical canal and the stratified squamous epithelium (left) that covers the vaginal surface of the cervix. Squamous epithelium has grown down into a cervical gland (centre), which is thus lined by a mixture of both types of epithelia. The squamous epithelium is normal, however, and the lesion is not neoplastic. The cervical canal (top) contains thick secretion. **12.31 and 12.32 Endocervical polyp.** **12.31** This benign lesion originates in the endocervix and its surface is covered with the mucin-secreting columnar cells characteristic of that site. The stroma of loose connective tissue contains large blood vessels but there is no evidence of chronic inflammation. **12.32** shows the characteristic tall mucin-secreting cells in more detail. They line the dilated and cystic glands within the polyp but on the surface (left) they have been replaced by flat non-mucin-secreting

cells. The surface is not ulcerated but the fibrous stroma is very vascular and infiltrated with chronic inflammatory cells. **12.33 Endometrial polyp.** Both the glandular elements and the stroma of this simple polyp are clearly of endometrial origin. The glands are non-secretory. The surface layer (left) of flattened epithelial cells is intact, there is no evidence of inflammation, and vascularity is slight. This lesion may be compared with 12.32 which is at the same magnification. **12.34 and 12.35 Carcinoma in situ: cervix.** **12.34** The stratified squamous epithelium is thicker than normal and the surface layers are keratinised. On the left the normal stratification has been preserved but in the lesion (right) the cell arrangement is haphazard and the nuclei are not only larger, more basophilic and more pleomorphic but also appear more 'crowded'. Higher-power examination would reveal greatly increased mitotic activity, with mitotic figures in all layers. The underlying tissues are vascular but lymphocytic infiltration is slight. **12.35** This shows in detail the malignant change in the cervical epithelium. The nuclei are large, pleomorphic and basophilic and there are mitotic figures (top left and top right) in the superficial layers. The architecture has been virtually destroyed though the most superficial cells are flattened and squamous. **12.36 Primary squamous carcinoma: cervix.** The tumour cells are very large and squamous and arranged in clumps which show characteristically no tendency to keratinisation. Mitotic activity was very moderate and no figures are present in this field. The stroma is scanty and infiltrated with lymphocytes.

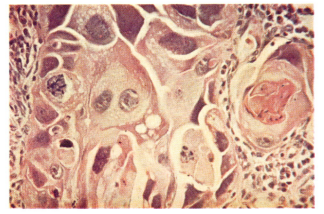

12.37 Primary squamous carcinoma: cervix

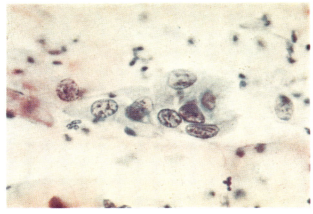

12.38 Primary squamous carcinoma: cervix

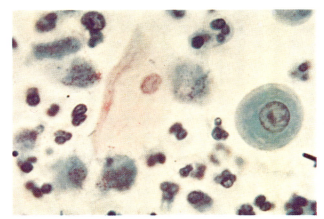

12.39 Trichomonas vaginalis: vaginal smear

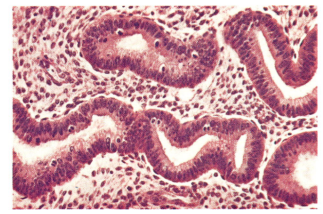

12.40 Proliferative phase: endometrium

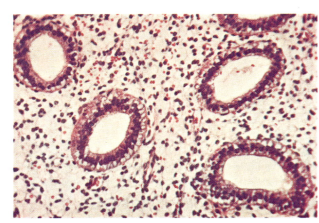

12.41 Early secretory phase: endometrium

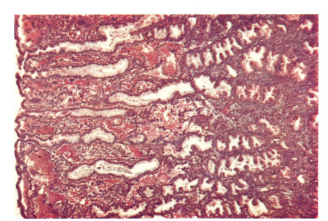

12.42 Premenstrual phase: endometrium

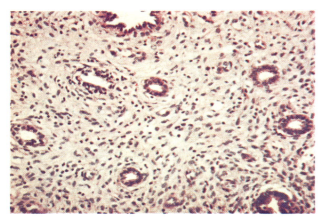

12.43 Contraceptive pill: endometrium

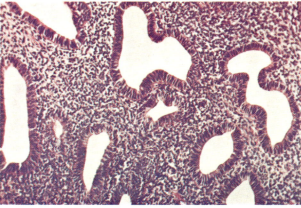

12.44 Non-secretory hyperplasia (metropathia haemor-rhagica): endometrium

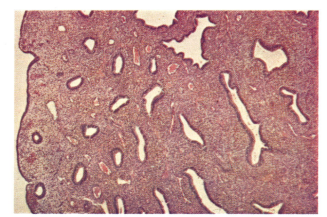

12.45 Post-menopause endometrium

12.37 and 12.38 Primary squamous carcinoma: cervix. 12.37 This is a biopsy taken some weeks after the tumour had been treated with x-rays. The cells are enormous and both cytoplasm and nucleus are swollen. The most striking change, however, is in the nuclear structure; that is, loss of the normal chromatin texture and partial or complete breakdown of nucleoli. The nuclear membrane is still intact. Plasma cells and lymphocytes infiltrate the stroma. **12.38** This is a vaginal smear. There is a cluster of squamous epithelial cells in the centre. Their nuclei show irregular distribution of chromatin, much of it being condensed on to the nuclear membrane. As a result the nuclear membrane varies in thickness from one place to another and areas of increased translucency have formed within the nucleus. The cytoplasm is scanty compared with the nuclear size. These features are highly suggestive of carcinoma. This patient had a squamous carcinoma of cervix confirmed by biopsy. **12.39 Trichomonas vaginalis.** This too is a vaginal smear stained by Papanicolaou's method. Seven Trichomonad organisms are present. Each has characteristic refractile magenta-coloured granules, a fuzzy outline, and a barely discernible nucleus. The parabasal epithelial cell (right) shows the nuclear changes characteristic of this infection. It has rounded up and the cytoplasm stains irregularly; and the chromatin has condensed on the nuclear membrane, leaving excessively pale areas. The deposition of chromatin is fairly even, whereas in a malignant cell the deposition is irregular. A large intermediate squamous epithelial cell is present (above centre) along with numerous pus cells. **12.40 Proliferative phase: endometrium.** The glands are lengthening and becoming sinuous in outline, and the epithelial cells, which tend to heap up, show intense mitotic activity. There is migration of the

nuclei towards the lumen of the gland prior to mitosis. Secretion has not yet begun. The stroma is becoming looser and more oedematous. **12.41 Early secretory phase: endometrium.** The glands are lined by a single layer of columnar epithelial cells. Beneath the nucleus of each cell is a large secretory vacuole. Vacuoles normally appear about the fourteenth day of the cycle. The stroma is very loose and oedematous. **12.42 Premenstrual phase: endometrium.** This low-power view shows large glands which in their deeper parts (right) have a dentate outline. The lumen (left) contains mucinous secretion. There is extensive haemorrhage into the superficial stroma and disintegration is already visible on the surface. **12.43 Contraceptive pill: endometrium.** The pill is a progestogen or a mixture of an oestrogen and a progestogen. The stroma shows a fairly well-developed pseudo-decidual reaction but the endometrial glands are small simple structures, lined by flattened or cuboidal hypoplastic non-secretory cells. **12.44 Non-secretory hyperplasia (metropathia haemorrhagica): endometrium.** The glands are moderately dilated and lined by a thick layer of hyperplastic epithelial cells. There is no evidence of secretion. The stroma is intensely cellular. Mitoses are present among both the epithelial and stromal cells. Elsewhere the glands were more dilated and cystic. **12.45 Post-menopause endometrium.** The post-menopausal endometrium is usually atrophic. In this example it is thicker than normal but the glands are widely separated and lined by columnar epithelium which shows no mitotic activity on higher power examination. The stroma is abundant, compact and rather fibrous. It is fairly vascular.

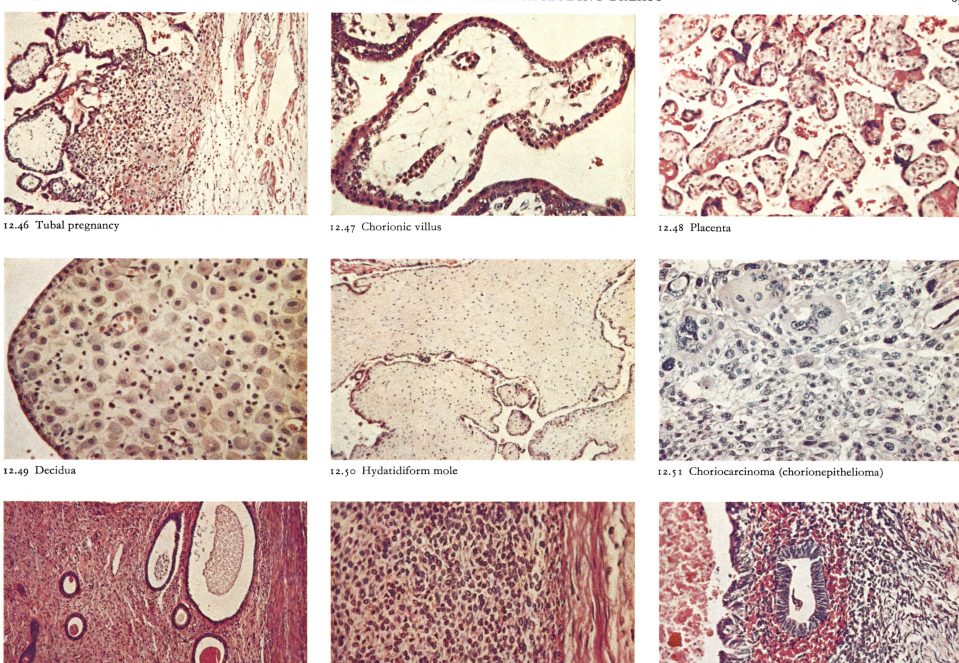

12.46 Tubal pregnancy

12.47 Chorionic villus

12.48 Placenta

12.49 Decidua

12.50 Hydatidiform mole

12.51 Choriocarcinoma (chorionepithelioma)

12.52 Adenomyosis: uterus

12.53 Stromatous endometriosis: uterus

12.54 Endometriosis: ovary

12.46 Tubal pregnancy. Thin-walled oedematous chorionic villi are present in the lumen of the tube (left). The cellular mass in the centre consists of cytotrophoblast and syncytiotrophoblast. The muscular wall of the tube (right) is thick and oedematous and a little haemorrhage has occurred. **12.47 Chorionic villus.** This shows a young (about 12 weeks) chorionic villus. The surface is covered by two layers of cells, the outer being the syncytiotrophoblast and the inner the cytotrophoblast. The core consists of stellate connective tissue cells and abundant intercellular substance which is unstained. The fetal blood vessels are packed with nucleated red cells. **12.48 Placenta.** This is a full-term placenta. These mature villi are smaller than young villi and the core is much more fibrous. Each has several fetal blood vessels. Most villi are covered with a single layer of syncytiotrophoblast nuclei but in many places the nuclei have proliferated and heaped up into basophilic masses. Fibrin deposition has occurred on the surface of many villi and in a few it has penetrated into the core. **12.49 Decidua.** The stromal cells are very swollen and have abundant, rather foamy cytoplasm which is rich in glycogen. These cells provide a rich medium for early growth and proliferation of the embryo before vascular development occurs. Intercellular oedema separates the decidual cells. The uterine cavity (left) is lined by cuboidal epithelium. **12.50 Hydatidiform mole.** The chorionic villi are large and cystic and the connective tissue cells of the core of the villi are widely separated by oedema fluid.

Fetal blood vessels are lacking. The degree of trophoblastic proliferation varies widely in moles. In this example it is slight. **12.51 Choriocarcinoma (chorionepithelioma).** This rare tumour may follow a normal pregnancy or an abortion. It may also follow hydatidiform mole. No villi are present and the tumour consists of cells derived from the cytotrophoblast (below) and syncytiotrophoblast (top). The tumour produces chorionic gonadotrophin and tests for this hormone are positive. **12.52 Adenomyosis: uterus.** The wall of the uterus was very thick and this is a section deep in the muscle coat (right). There is a nodule lying in the myometrium which consists of glands and stroma clearly of endometrial origin. Some glands contain secretion but there is no evidence of previous haemorrhage in or around the lesion. The stroma is fairly fibrous. The islands of endometrial tissue are in direct continuity with the endometrium lining the uterus. **12.53 Stromatous endometriosis: uterus.** A compact and well-circumscribed mass of cells (left) which closely resemble the stromal cells of proliferative phase endometrium is present within the myometrium (right). It is not accompanied by glandular elements and there is no evidence of haemorrhage. The exact nature and origin of this rare lesion is still a matter for debate. **12.54 Endometriosis: ovary.** Endometrial glands and stroma are present on the surface of the ovary and there is evidence of haemorrhage, both old and recent, in their vicinity.

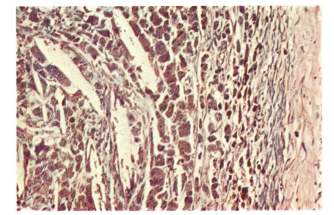

12.55 Endometriosis: ovary

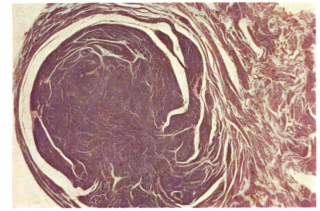

12.56 Leiomyoma: uterus

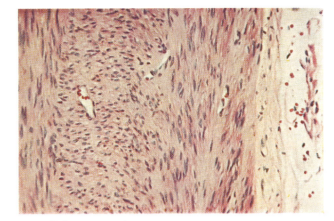

12.57 Leiomyoma: uterus

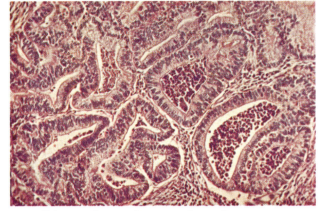

12.58 Primary adenocarcinoma: endometrium

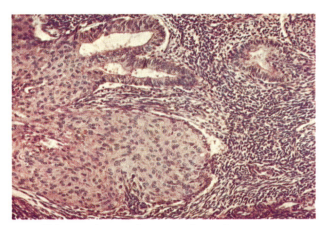

12.59 Primary adenocarcinoma: endometrium

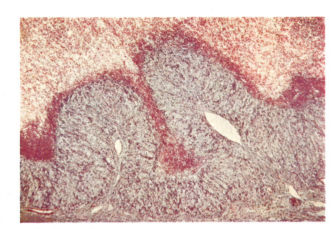

12.60 Corpus luteum cyst

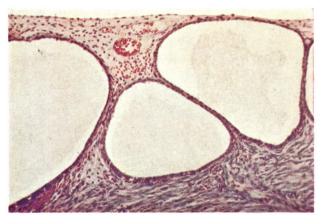

12.61 Germinal inclusion cysts: ovary

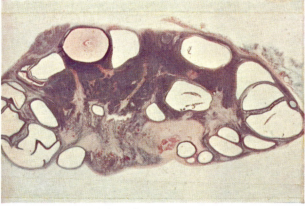

12.62 Stein-Leventhal syndrome: ovary

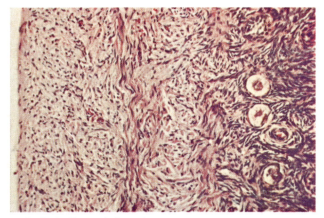

12.63 Stein-Leventhal syndrome: ovary

12.55 Endometriosis: ovary. This shows the reaction that has occurred to the haemorrhage around the endometrial elements. The red cells have been digested by macrophages and most of the cells here are lipofuscin-laden phagocytes. Fibrous tissue has also formed (right). The clefts were occupied by cholesterol crystals which are often found in old haemorrhages. **12.56** and **12.57 Leiomyoma: uterus. 12.56** Though the tumour (left) is rounded and well-demarcated from the muscle coat (right) of the uterus, it has no capsule. It consists of interlacing bands of smooth muscle and a small amount of fibrous tissue. Being more cellular than the uterine muscle it is more basophilic. **12.57** This shows in detail the well-defined edge of the tumour and the lack of a definite capsule. The neoplasm is benign and consists of mature smooth-muscle cells. These form bundles which run at various angles so that some are seen in longitudinal section and some in cross-section. There is a little fibrous tissue lying between the muscle fibrils and this usually increases so that older tumours often become very hard and fibrous. **12.58** and **12.59 Primary adenocarcinoma: endometrium. 12.58** This is part of the bulky tissue that filled the uterine cavity. It is adenocarcinomatous and consists of very abnormal and closely-packed glands whose 'back to back' arrangement is noteworthy. There is considerable mitotic activity in the columnar epithelial cells forming these glands and some glands contain cell debris. The

stroma is scanty. **12.59** A well-differentiated adenocarcinoma (top) is invading the myometrium (right). In some areas the glandular elements are replaced by masses of squamous epithelium (left) that does not look unduly malignant. Lesions showing this change are sometimes termed adeno-acanthomas. **12.60 Corpus luteum cyst.** The wall of the cyst consists of granulosa lutein and theca lutein. The cyst appears to be the result of massive haemorrhage (above) into the centre of a corpus luteum. **12.61 Germinal inclusion cysts: ovary.** These are simple cysts lined by cuboidal or flattened epithelium derived from the so-called germinal epithelium on the surface of the ovary (top). Their watery contents are pale-staining. **12.62** and **12.63 Stein-Leventhal syndrome: ovary.** In this syndrome there is amenorrhoea and hirsutism, in combination with enlarged and cystic ovaries. **12.62** This ovary (5 cm. long) is from a patient aged 18 years. The enlargement is due to the presence of many cystic follicles. Higher-power examination of these follicles showed the presence of a hypertrophied theca interna which had undergone luteinisation. However ovulation does not occur and there are no corpora lutea or corpora albicantes. The superficial cortex is fibrous. **12.63** The surface of the ovary is fibrotic and some of the ova (right) are degenerate.

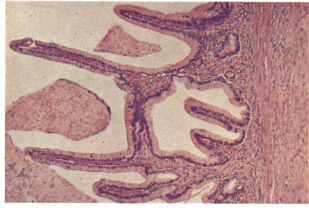

12.64 Mucinous cystadenoma: ovary

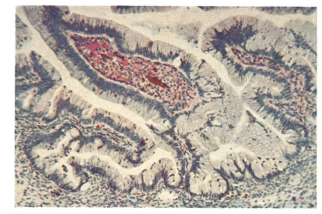

12.65 Mucinous cystadenocarcinoma: ovary

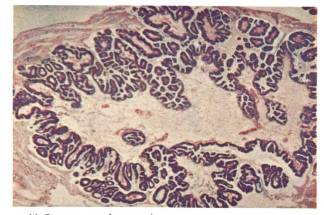

12.66 Serous cystadenocarcinoma: ovary

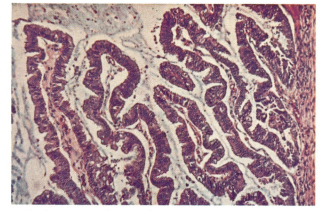

12.67 Serous cystadenocarcinoma: ovary

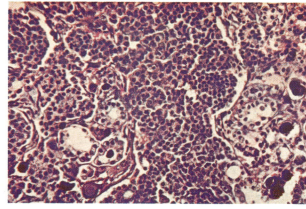

12.68 Serous cystadenocarcinoma: ovary

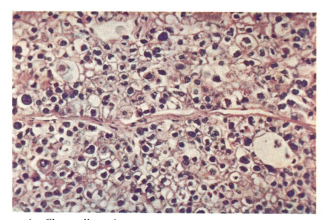

12.69 Clear cell carcinoma: ovary

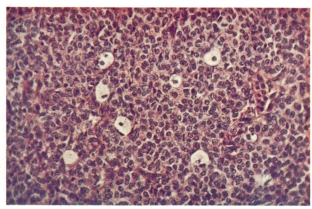

12.70 Granulosa cell tumour: ovary

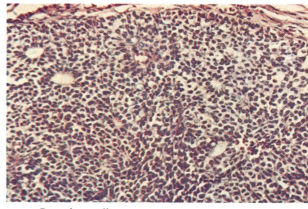

12.71 Granulosa cell tumour: ovary

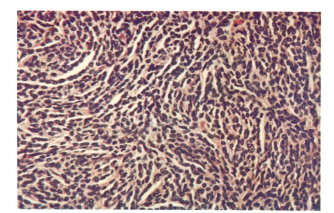

12.72 Granulosa cell tumour: ovary

12.64 Mucinous cystadenoma: ovary. This tumour often grows to a large size and is filled with thick mucoid fluid. The cyst has a thick fibrous wall (right) lined by columnar epithelium which forms papilliform ingrowths. The epithelial cells are structurally similar to endocervical epithelium and secrete the mucin, some of which is still visible in the lumen. **12.65 Mucinous cystadenocarcinoma: ovary.** Numerous papilliform processes project into the lumen. The tumour cells are very large and secrete abundant mucin. Their nuclei are also large and basophilic and mitotic activity was fairly marked on high power examination. However the degree of malignancy is moderate. The wall is fibrous. **12.66–12.68 Serous cystadenocarcinoma: ovary. 12.66** This is part of a large cystic tumour that was filled with watery fluid. The structure is papilliferous and the cells are large and basophilic. Mucin secretion is not a feature. **12.67** This shows the papilliform processes of the tumour in more detail. Their stroma is delicate and the covering epithelium consists of tall columnar cells which exhibit considerable mitotic activity. **12.68** This is a more solid part of another serous cystadenocarcinoma. The tumour cells form sheets and irregular acini. Scattered irregularly throughout the neoplastic tissue are small spherical calcified masses (psammoma bodies). The epithelium of serous and mucinous cystadenomas and cystadenocarcinomas is derived from the germinal epithelium of the ovary. **12.69 Clear cell carcinoma: ovary.** The cells are polyhedral and have abundant 'clear' cytoplasm and resemble those of renal carcinoma. Although nuclear hyperchromatism and pleomorphism are prominent, no mitoses are present in this field. Stroma is very scanty. **12.70–12.72 Granulosa cell tumour: ovary.** Granulosa cell tumours vary widely in histological structure, and range from the pure granulosa cell tumour with few thecal elements through thecomas to luteinomas. Granulosa cell tumours have marked oestrogenic (feminising) effects. **12.70** This specimen consists entirely of closely-packed polyhedral granulosa cells which show a tendency to form follicles (Call-Exner bodies). **12.71** The granulosa cells have a folliculoid pattern and several Call-Exner bodies are present. **12.72** In this specimen the cells have little cytoplasm and are arranged in long cords.

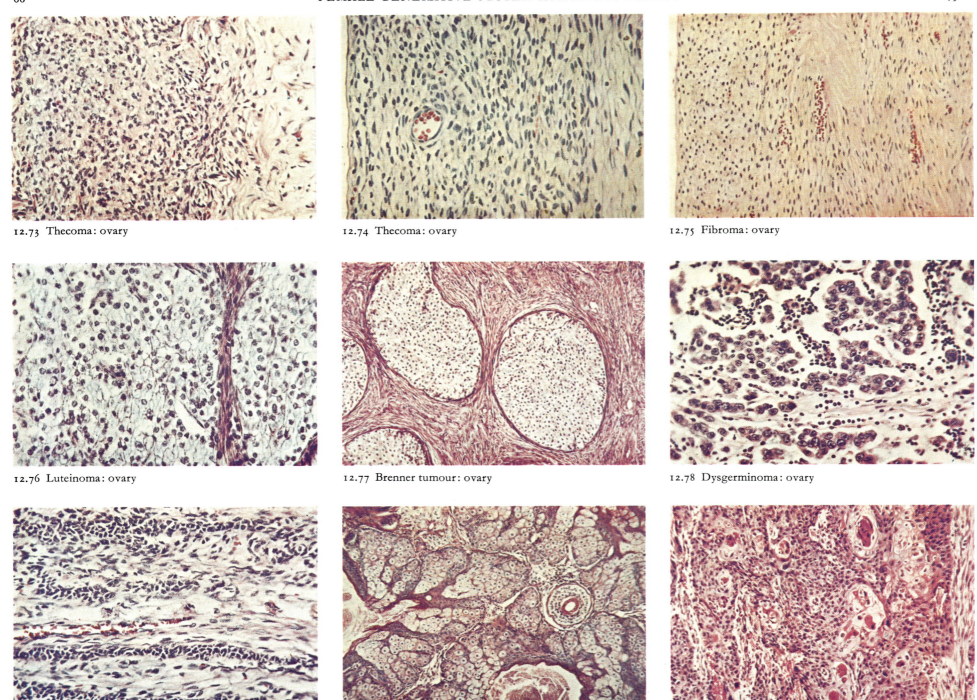

12.73 Thecoma: ovary

12.74 Thecoma: ovary

12.75 Fibroma: ovary

12.76 Luteinoma: ovary

12.77 Brenner tumour: ovary

12.78 Dysgerminoma: ovary

12.79 Arrhenoblastoma: ovary

12.80 Benign cystic teratoma (dermoid cyst): ovary

12.81 Benign cystic teratoma of ovary: malignant change

12.73 and **12.74 Thecoma: ovary. 12.73** In one part of the tumour (right) the cells are fibroblastic and the tissue around them is fibrous and collagenous. In the other part of the tumour (left) the cells are more numerous, have plump oval nuclei, many seen on cross-section. A silver stain would show reticulin fibres surrounding the individual cells. **12.74** This is the periphery of a tumour that was generally more fibrous than 12.73. The cells look like young fibroblasts and possess ovoid nuclei and around them is abundant collagen. It is often difficult to distinguish between a fibrous thecoma and a fibroma of ovary. The presence of neutral fat droplets in the thecoma sometimes helps. **12.75 Fibroma: ovary.** The tumour consists of interlacing bundles of collagenous fibrous connective tissue which shows a tendency to become hyalinised. **12.76 Luteinoma: ovary.** In this form of granulosa cell tumour the cells resemble the lutein cells of the mature corpus luteum and like them are yellow macroscopically, because of their abundant lipid. Microscopically, as here, they are large and have abundant granular (lipid-rich) cytoplasm. A band of fibrous stroma is present. **12.77 Brenner tumour: ovary.** Large 'nests' of epithelial cells which resemble transitional or squamous epithelium lie in a dense fibrous stroma. This is a benign tumour of doubtful histogenesis. **12.78 Dysgerminoma: ovary.** The

tumour cells are large and resemble the primordial germ cells of the sexually indifferent embryonic gonad and the tumour is morphologically identical with the seminoma. The cells are arranged in groups and cords and show some nuclear pleomorphism. No mitoses are present in this field, but there were scattered figures elsewhere in the tumour. The stroma is fibrous and delicate and contains many lymphocytes. The spaces are the result of processing shrinkage. **12.79 Arrhenoblastoma: ovary.** The basophilic tumour cells form long cords which resemble primitive seminiferous tubules. Interstitial cells are sometimes present, though none are present in this tumour's stroma. The arrhenoblastoma usually produces defeminisation and masculinisation. **12.80** and **12.81 Benign cystic teratoma (dermoid cyst): ovary. 12.80** The specimen was a unilocular cyst full of sebaceous material and hair. This part of the wall consists of sebaceous glands which open into numerous ducts. A hair follicle can also be seen (right of centre). A variety of other tissues, fully differentiated, was present elsewhere in the wall. **12.81** Malignant change has taken place in the epithelial element of this teratoma and a squamous cell carcinoma has resulted. It is a well-differentiated tumour forming fairly abundant keratin. Some of the tumour cell nuclei are large and very basophilic.

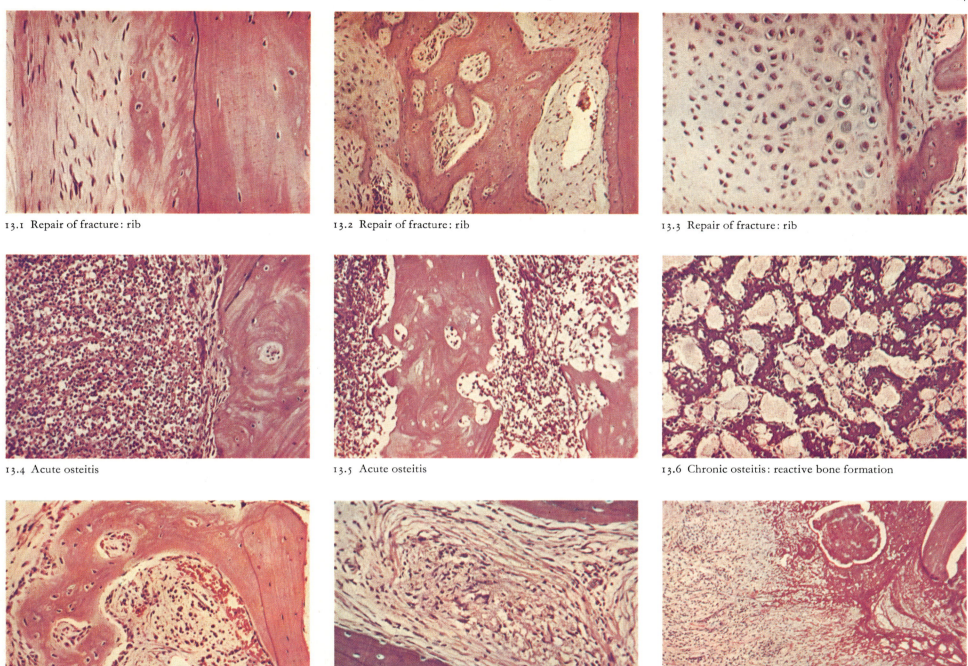

13.1 Repair of fracture: rib

13.2 Repair of fracture: rib

13.3 Repair of fracture: rib

13.4 Acute osteitis

13.5 Acute osteitis

13.6 Chronic osteitis: reactive bone formation

13.7 Chronic osteitis: reactive bone formation

13.8 Tuberculosis: bone

13.9 Tuberculosis: bone

13.1-13.3 Repair of fracture: rib. 13.1 The periosteum adjacent to the fracture is reacting. It has become thicker and three layers can be distinguished. First, a fibrous layer (left) resembling normal 'resting' periosteum; secondly a zone of potential osteoblasts, and thirdly a layer (centre) of newly-formed woven (coarse-fibred) bone. A cement line separates the new bone from the lamellar bone of the rib cortex (right). The lamellar bone osteocytes are flat and arranged parallel to the surface. The blue dots in the bone matrix are their numerous cytoplasmic processes. The woven bone osteocytes are more rounded and less regularly arranged. Woven bone is a more primitive form of bone than lamellar bone. It is basophilic and chemically not unlike hyaline cartilage. It is usually replaced by lamellar bone. **13.2** A thick layer of external callus has formed on the surface of the cortical bone (right) adjacent to the fracture. The callus consists of vascular connective tissue, thick trabeculae of woven bone (centre) and hyaline cartilage (left) Active-looking osteoblasts cover the surfaces of the newly-formed bone. **13.3** This is internal callus filling the gap between the bone ends. It has the same structure as the external callus, consisting of cellular hyaline cartilage (centre and left) and trabeculae of woven bone (right). Osteoblasts cover the surfaces of the bone trabeculae and cellular connective tissue fills the spaces between them. **13.4 and 13.5 Acute osteitis. 13.4** The marrow (left) is full of pus. The pus consists largely of neutrophil polymorphs, though macrophages are fairly numerous. The bone trabeculae (right) are being eroded but the presence of osteocytes in the lacunae shows that the bone is alive. **13.5** Erosion is here much more extensive. It would appear that enzymes are

released from the pus cells which can digest the bone trabeculae, perhaps only when they are necrotic. Most of the osteocyte lacunae are empty and the bone appears to be dead. **13.6 and 13.7 Chronic osteitis: reactive bone formation.** This shows reactive bone formation in the vicinity of a chronic pyogenic inflammatory lesion. **13.6** The new bone consists of intensely basophilic interlacing trabeculae of woven bone. They lie in delicate connective tissue, from which they have formed by 'ossification in membrane'. **13.7** The normal haemopoietic marrow has been replaced by vascular connective tissue (below centre) which contains a moderate number of plasma cells and lymphocytes. The bone on the right is normal lamellar bone but on its surface new woven bone has formed (top and left). The surface of this new bone is covered with large active osteoblasts. A prominent cement line marks the junction between the two types of bone. **13.8 and 13.9 Tuberculosis: bone. 13.8** A large follicle lies between two lamellar bone trabeculae. The follicle consists of epithelioid cells and giant cells. There is evidence of repair and at the periphery fibroblasts, perhaps derived from the epithelioid cells, are forming a fibrous tissue capsule. **13.9** This is a much more destructive lesion than 13.8. The bone trabecula (top right) is necrotic and its osteocyte lacunae are empty. The tissue on the left is tuberculous granulation tissue, rich in macrophages, lymphocytes and epithelioid cells but containing relatively few capillaries. There are no follicles. Between this tissue and the bone trabecula there is deeply eosinophilic necrotic tissue which was caseous on macroscopic examination.

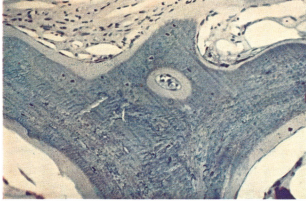

13.10 Osteomalacia

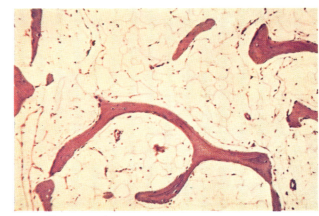

13.11 Osteoporosis

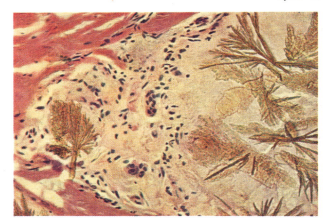

13.12 Gout

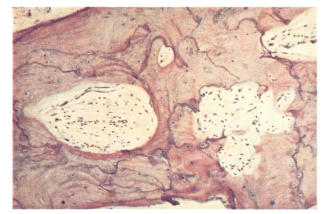

13.13 Paget's disease (osteitis deformans): skull

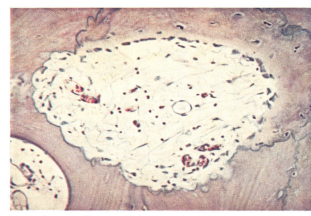

13.14 Paget's disease: skull

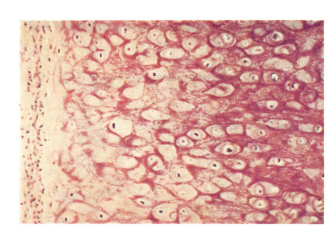

13.15 Necrosis (post-irradiation): cartilage

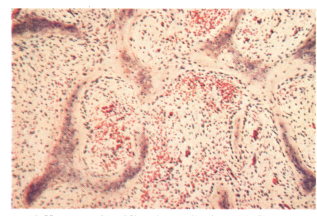

13.16 Hyperparathyroidism (generalised osteitis fibrosa cystica): bone

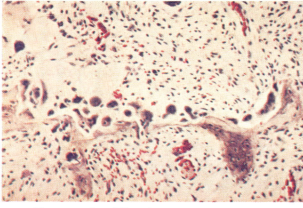

13.17 Hyperparathyroidism: bone

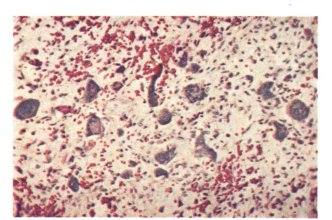

13.18 Hyperparathyroidism: bone

13.10 Osteomalacia. In osteomalacia the bones are soft because of defective mineralisation. In this example the bone has not been decalcified during processing and the bone salts stain heavily with haematoxylin. The non-calcified layer of osteoid on the surface of the trabecula is unstained. It is wider than normal. The marrow (above) is characteristically fibrous. **13.11 Osteoporosis.** Osteoporosis means rarefaction of the bone as a result of loss of protein matrix. The trabeculae are thin and delicate and widely separated by fatty marrow. There is no evidence of deficient calcification, however, and the osteoid seams seen in osteomalacia are lacking. The osteoblasts on the surface of the trabeculae are flat and inactive-looking. There is no osteoclastic activity. **13.12 Gout:** This is a tophus. It consists of collections of amorphous and crystalline sodium biurate which have provoked a macrophage and giant cell reaction, as well as considerable fibrosis. **13.13 and 13.14 Paget's disease (osteitis deformans): skull. 13.13** The trabeculae are very irregular and thick. Running through them is a 'mosaic' of blue cement lines which are evidence of many previous episodes of patchy bone resorption and deposition. The notching of the trabeculae should be noted. Despite their thickness the trabeculae are not strong and separate readily at the cement lines. Cellular connective tissue fills the spaces between the bone trabeculae. **13.14** This shows in more detail the irregular curved cement lines (right and top) which form the charac-

teristic mosaic and the vascular connective tissue that fills the marrow spaces. Osteoblasts are laying down new bone on one side (top) whereas on the other side (bottom) the notching of the lamellar bone trabeculae suggests very strongly that resorption is occurring, even though osteoclasts are not visible. **13.15 Necrosis (post-irradiation): cartilage.** Though the cells of the perichondrium (left) appear to be unaffected the chondrocytes are probably all necrotic. Many have no nuclei and others have nuclei that stain weakly or not at all. Moreover the matrix has lost its characteristic basophilia and stains red. Necrosis of cartilage is a troublesome complication of x-ray therapy. **13.16–13.18 Hyperparathyroidism (generalised osteitis fibrosa cystica): bone. 13.16** The normal bone has been replaced by a vascular and cellular connective tissue within which basophilic trabeculae of woven bone are forming by 'ossification in membrane'. Some of these trabeculae have fairly broad pink osteoid seams and are probably poorly calcified. There is fairly extensive haemorrhage. **13.17** In this zone there is very active resorption of bone by osteoclasts. The bone appears to be of woven type and only recently formed in the vascular connective tissue. **13.18** Cellular connective tissue rich in osteoclasts, as shown here, is often present in large amounts within the affected bones. Haemorrhage into this tissue occurs readily and colours it brown, and it may come to resemble closely a giant cell tumour of bone.

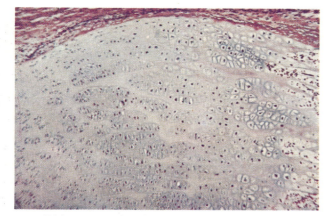

13.19 Rickets: costochondral junction

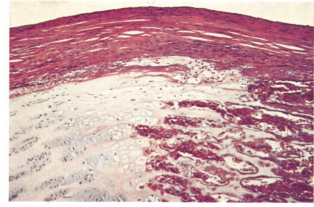

13.20 Rickets: costochondral junction

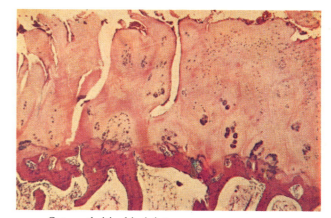

13.21 Osteoarthritis: hip-joint

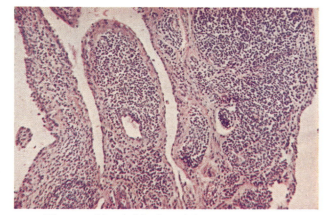

13.22 Rheumatoid arthritis: knee-joint

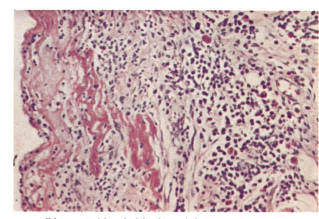

13.23 Rheumatoid arthritis: knee-joint

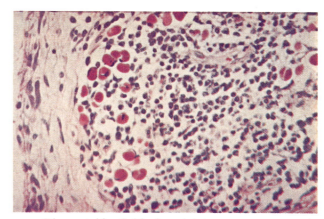

13.24 Rheumatoid arthritis: knee-joint

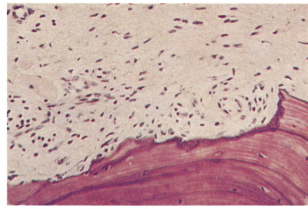

13.25 Rheumatoid arthritis: metacarpo-phalangeal joint

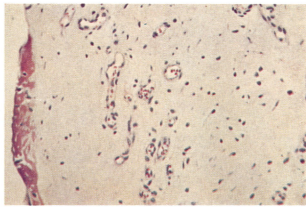

13.26 Rheumatoid arthritis: tendon sheath

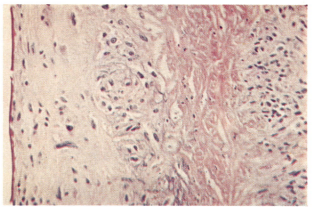

13.27 Rheumatoid arthritis: tendon sheath

13.19 and **13.20 Rickets: costo-chondral junction. 13.19** The cartilage matrix in the zone of hypertrophic cells has failed to calcify. As a result, the normal maturation of the chondrocytes, with their eventual death, does not occur. Instead of slim columns of cells neatly piled one on top of the other, the chondrocytes form very broad irregular columns, so that the epiphysis is enlarged and bulges. Moreover the blood vessels growing up from the metaphysis fail to digest and remove the matrix, probably because living cartilage is more difficult to digest than dead cartilage. **13.20** This shows a similar lesion, thick columns of irregularly-arranged chondrocytes and a bulging epiphysis. The metaphyseal vessels are prominent, as they attempt to erode the matrix between the columns of hypertrophied and fully viable cartilage cells. A considerable amount of matrix, still not calcified, survives in the trabeculae of newly-formed bone. **13.21 Osteoarthritis: hip-joint.** The articular cartilage covering the bone is fibrillated, and deep clefts have formed in it. Clusters of chondrocytes remain but many of these cells have disappeared, leaving acellular matrix. Some of the chondrocytes in the clusters are large and hypertrophic. **13.22–13.24 Rheumatoid arthritis: knee-joint. 13.22** Villi of proliferated synovial tissue project into the joint space. These processes consist of connective tissue covered with flattened fibroblast-like synovial cells and are heavily infiltrated with plasma cells and lymphocytes. **13.23** This is a higher power view of the lesion in 13.22. In the surface layers of the synovial tissue are collec-

tions of deeply eosinophilic 'fibrinoid' material. Some of this is probably fibrin but probably some is necrotic connective tissue ('fibrinoid necrosis'). Plasma cells and Russell bodies (swollen eosinophilic plasma cells) are numerous in the deeper layers. **13.24** This shows in more detail the synovial lining cells and the cellular infiltrate which consists almost wholly of plasma cells. The Russell bodies are prominent. In them the nucleus is greatly compressed. **13.25 Rheumatoid arthritis.** This is from an ankylosed metacarpo-phalangeal joint. It shows (top) a small part of the connective tissue (pannus) that had grown across the surface of the head of the metacarpal bone (bottom) to fill the joint space. The articular cartilage which covered the metacarpal has been destroyed and only a few loose fragments remain. **13.26** and **13.27 Rheumatoid arthritis: tendon sheath. 13.26** Here the connective tissue of the sheath is very vascular and oedematous and there are scattered lymphocytes. On the lining surface is a small plaque of fibrin. This is a very early stage, and it is possible that trauma alone could produce a mild tenosynovitis of this degree. **13.27** Here too, a thin layer of fibrin has formed on the lining surface. However in the fibrous wall of the tendon sheath there is also a characteristic nodule, consisting of a necrotic centre surrounded by macrophages. Slight palisading of these cells is present but it is usually much more pronounced.

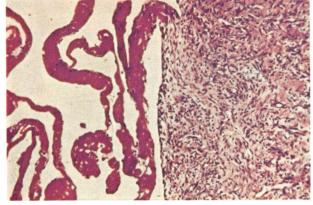

13.28 Olecranon bursitis

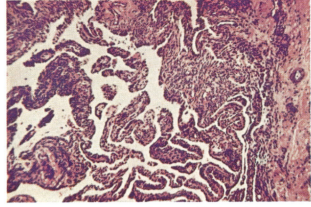

13.29 Pigmented villo-nodular synovitis: knee joint

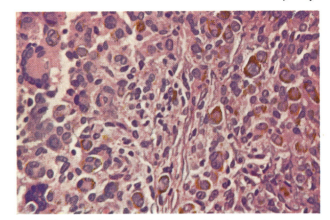

13.30 Pigmented villo-nodular synovitis: knee joint

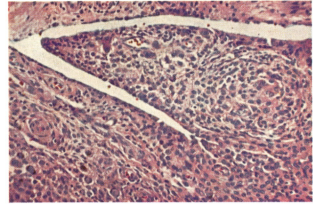

13.31 Giant cell tumour of tendon sheath (benign synovioma)

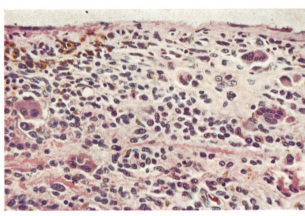

13.32 Giant cell tumour of tendon sheath

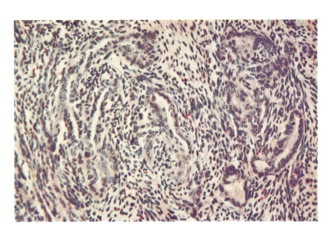

13.33 Synovial sarcoma (synovioma)

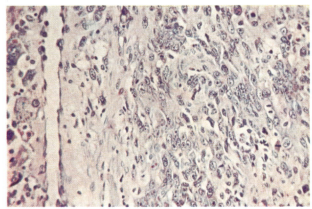

13.34 Synovial sarcoma

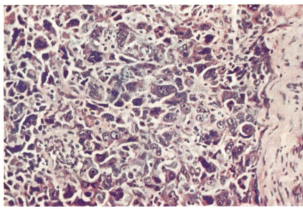

13.35 Synovial sarcoma

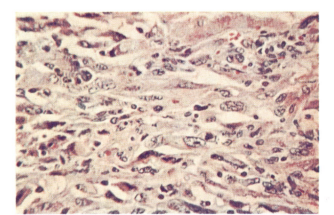

13.36 Alveolar soft-part sarcoma

13.28 Olecranon bursitis. The wall of the bursa (right) is thick and fibrous and lined by flattened synovial cells (centre). There is mild lymphocytic infiltration of the fibrous tissue. Within the bursal sac (left) and attached to the wall are long dense strands and coils of fibrin. This lesion is usually the result of trauma. **13.29** and **13.30 Pigmented villo-nodular synovitis: knee-joint. 13.29** Characteristically it is the knee-joint that is affected. Large numbers of villi project from the capsule (right) into the joint. These villi are fibrous and vascular but lack the intense lymphocytic and plasma cell population found in a rheumatoid lesion. **13.30** is a higher power view of the proliferating synovial tissue. It is intensely cellular and the closely-packed cells show a variety of forms and have ill-defined boundaries. Some are multinucleate. Many are laden with haemosiderin. These appearances are very similar to that seen in the giant cell tumour of tendon sheath (benign synovioma). **13.31** and **13.32 Giant cell tumour of tendon sheath (benign synovioma). 13.31** The synovial sheath is at the top. The lesion consists of closely-packed cells that range from spindle-shaped fibroblasts to multinucleate phagocytes. **13.32** Higher power examination shows the multinucleate character of many of the cells. There is a considerable amount of fibrous intercellular material and extracellular haemosiderin is also present (top left). The multinucleate cells do not contain haemosiderin but elsewhere many were full of pigment

and resembled those shown in 13.30. The distinction between giant cell tumour of tendon sheath and villo-nodular synovitis is often a matter of opinion and of the affected site. **13.33–13.35 Synovial sarcoma. 13.33** The tumour cells are spindle-shaped with dark-staining nuclei, and a considerable amount of fibrous intercellular material is present. The cells tend to form clefts and as often happens the cells lining the clefts have altered to resemble glandular epithelium. **13.34** In this tumour the cells are large and exhibit considerable mitotic activity (right) and the nucleoli are particularly prominent. The cells still exhibit a tendency to form clefts (left) lined by flattened cells. **13.35** This is an even more active tumour than the previous one and the extremely pleomorphic nuclei have multiple nucleoli. There are many mitoses. A fibrous tissue capsule is present round this part of the tumour (right) but it was deficient elsewhere. Synovial sarcomas are generally highly malignant. **13.36 Alveolar soft-part sarcoma.** The tumour is composed of very large elongated cells with irregular nuclei in which there are prominent nucleoli. Each cell has abundant granular cytoplasm. Some of the nuclei are pyknotic but there are no mitoses. This lesion is somewhat atypical. Usually the neoplastic cells are grouped into well-defined 'nests' or alveoli.

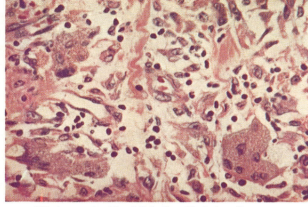

13.37 Histiocytosis: Hand-Schüller-Christian disease

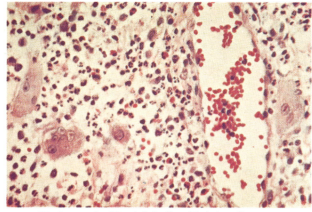

13.38 Histiocytosis: Hand-Schüller-Christian disease

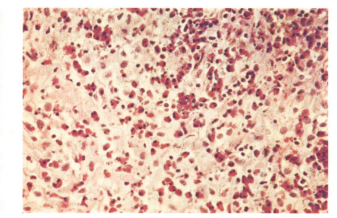

13.39 Histiocytosis: eosinophilic granuloma of bone

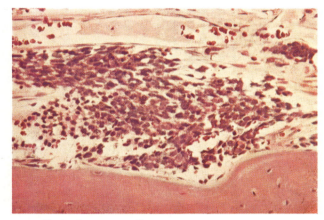

13.40 Ewing's sarcoma: femur

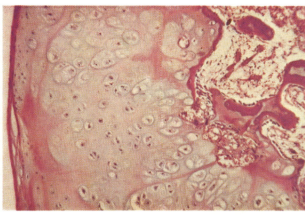

13.41 Osteochondroma (cartilaginous exostosis): femur

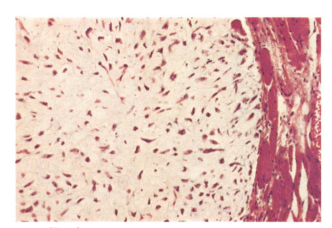

13.42 Chondrosarcoma

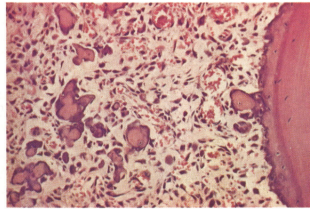

13.43 Osteosarcoma: femur

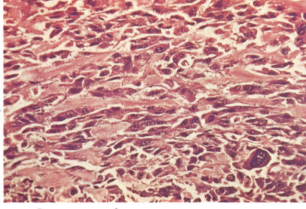

13.44 Osteosarcoma: femur

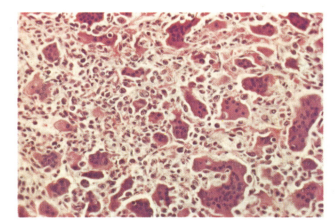

13.45 Giant cell tumour (osteoclastoma): fibula

13.37–13.39 Histiocytosis. 13.37 and 13.38 Hand-Schüller-Christian disease: bone. 13.37 The lesion consists of macrophages, many multinucleate, with abundant granular cytoplasm, lymphocytes and fibrous tissue. The lipid distending the phagocytes and causing the granular appearance of their cytoplasm consists of cholesterol esters. Wherever it forms the new tissue destroys the bone and the clinical picture depends on the sites of deposition. **13.38** In this deposit there are, in addition to the characteristic multinucleated foamy giant cells, many polymorph leucocytes. A high proportion of these are eosinophils and when eosinophils greatly predominate, the lesion resembles an 'eosinophilic granuloma' of bone. **13.39 Eosinophilic granuloma: bone.** This lesion is usually solitary and benign but destructive. The tissue replacing the marrow consists of eosinophils and large macrophages with abundant granular (lipid-rich) cytoplasm. Hand-Schüller-Christian disease and eosinophilic granuloma are examples of abnormal lipid storage. Letterer-Siwe disease is probably a third member of the same group. It is the most malignant and lipid storage is usually not a feature. **13.40 Ewing's sarcoma: femur.** This shows the tissue that filled the medullary cavity. It consists of a compact mass of cells with basophilic nuclei and little cytoplasm, characteristically accompanied by a highly vascular loose connective tissue. This uncommon tumour of children probably arises from the reticular tissue of the bone marrow. It may well be confused with metastatic neuroblastoma. It destroys bone but does not form it. The bone at the bottom is cortical bone. **13.41 Osteochondroma (cartilaginous exostosis).** This was a small hard sessile mass attached to the shaft of the femur near the knee-joint. It consists of mature bone (right) capped with cartilage (left). On the surface (left) there is a thin

layer of fibrous tissue which acts as a perichondrium and is continuous with the periosteum of the femur. New bone is formed 'in cartilage' by erosion of the deep aspect of the cartilage by capillary blood vessels in the same way as epiphysial cartilage is eroded in normal bone growth. **13.42 Chondrosarcoma.** This is the growing edge of the tumour. The cells are stellate and embedded in abundant mucopolysaccharide-rich basophilic matrix, the tissue being more myxomatous than cartilaginous. There is no perichondrium and the striated muscle (right) is being invaded on a broad front. The tumour compresses the muscle fibres but does not send slender columns of cells infiltrating between the fibrils. **13.43 and 13.44 Osteosarcoma: femur. 13.43** The sarcoma cells closely resemble osteoblasts and are forming much pale-staining osteoid. The tumour is destroying normal lamellar bone (right) and the small islands of bone within the tumour are probably surviving remnants of this bone. The blood vessels are thin-walled and apparently incompletely lined by endothelium. **13.44** In this lesion the cells are very large and elongated and have pleomorphic nuclei. They have formed a considerable amount of homogeneous pink osteoid. **13.45 Giant cell tumour (osteoclastoma).** This tumour, which characteristically occurs at the ends of long bones, was in the head of the fibula. It consists of a cellular 'stroma' of sarcoma-like tissue and numerous multinucleated giant cells resembling osteoclasts. The connective tissue element does not form osteoid or bone but it is actively growing and the tumour is very destructive locally. Up to a quarter of these tumours metastasise. Haemorrhage into the tumour is frequent and the lesion is usually red or dark brown in colour.

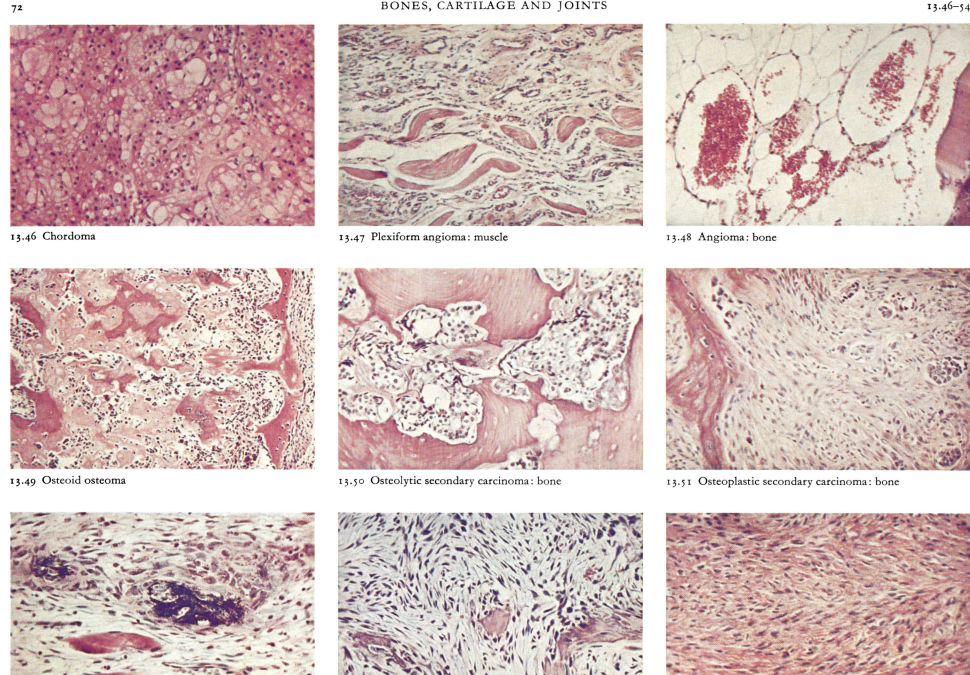

13.46 Chordoma

13.47 Plexiform angioma: muscle

13.48 Angioma: bone

13.49 Osteoid osteoma

13.50 Osteolytic secondary carcinoma: bone

13.51 Osteoplastic secondary carcinoma: bone

13.52 Progressive myositis ossificans

13.53 Polyostotic fibrous dysplasia (Albright's syndrome)

13.54 Dupuytren's contracture

13.46 Chordoma. The lesion, which arises from the notochord, was situated in the sacrococcygeal region. Many of the cells are large, with vacuolated cytoplasm (physaliferous cells). In places a great deal of extracellular mucoid material is present (bottom right, for example). The nuclei are mostly small and regular in form, though a few are rather larger. **13.47 Plexiform angioma: muscle.** The lesion consists of large numbers of arterioles and small venules lying among atrophic striated muscle fibres. **13.48 Angioma: bone.** In the fatty marrow between the bone trabeculae there are thin-walled blood vessels. These vessels, by increasing in number and expanding, may cause great destruction of bone. **13.49 Osteoid osteoma.** This was a painful lesion in the head of the ulna. The lesion consists of irregular masses of pink-staining osteoid and basophilic bone. Dark-staining osteoblasts are very numerous in the vascular connective tissue surrounding the osteoid and bone trabeculae. Part of the fibrous capsule that was present is visible on the right. **13.50 Osteolytic secondary carcinoma.** This is a secondary deposit of an adenocarcinoma of prostate in a vertebral body. The tumour cells, which form imperfect acini, are eroding the trabeculae of lamellar bone. The nuclei of the osteocytes stain very poorly and the bone is probably necrotic. **13.51 Osteoplastic secondary carcinoma.** This too is a deposit of prostatic carcinoma in a vertebral body. However in this case the marrow has been replaced by cellular connective tissue in which trabeculae of woven bone are forming (left). Formation of the connective tissue and bone has apparently been induced by the tumour cells visible as compact clusters on the right. Most prostatic metastases are osteosclerotic. **13.52 Progressive myositis ossificans.** A richly cellular, rather myxoid, connective tissue (above) has spread through the muscles (below). Groups of cells in this tissue have enlarged and differentiated into osteoblasts which have formed pink osteoid and blue-staining (calcified) bone. The bone thus formed 'in membrane' is 'woven' (coarse-fibred) bone. **13.53 Polyostotic fibrous dysplasia (Albright's syndrome).** The bone medulla has been expanded by a loosely-textured connective tissue, rich in elongated or stellate fibroblasts. These cells are tending by enlarging and acquiring more basophilic cytoplasm (top) to turn into osteoblasts and form trabeculae of woven bone (bottom). These spicules of bone are characteristically curved or sickle-shaped. The bone is poorly formed and resorption occurs readily. The precise nature of Albright's syndrome is debatable. In addition to the bone lesions which tend to be unilateral, the syndrome is characterised by patchy brown (café-au-lait) pigmentation of the skin, usually on the same side as the bone lesions, and endocrine disturbances including precocious puberty in the female. Monostotic fibrous dysplasia, not linked with Albright's syndrome, affects only one bone. **13.54 Dupuytren's contracture.** This lesion results from proliferation of elongated fibroblasts in the palmar fascia which form large amounts of fibrous tissue. This fibrous tissue replaces the fatty tissues of the region as well as the adjacent skin appendages. As the collagenous tissue matures and contracts, it produces the characteristic deformity of the palmar fascia and flexion of the fingers.

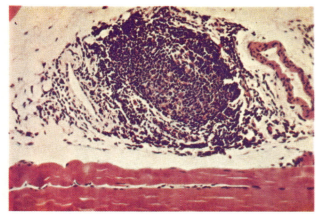

13.55 Rheumatoid arthritis: muscle

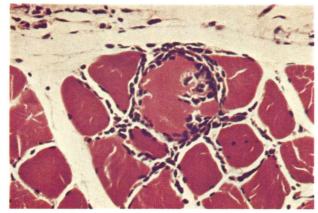

13.56 Rheumatoid arthritis: muscle

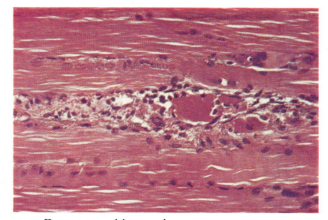

13.57 Dermatomyositis: muscle

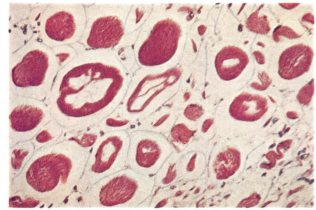

13.58 Dermatomyositis: muscle

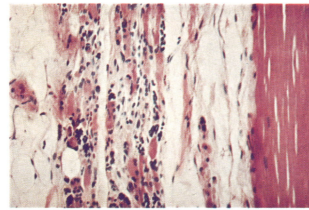

13.59 Neurogenic atrophy: muscle

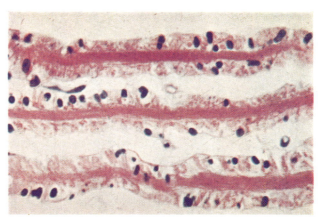

13.60 Neurogenic atrophy: muscle

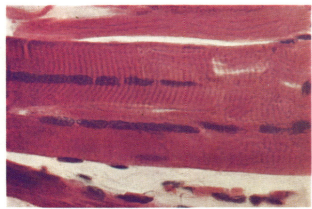

13.61 Myotonic dystrophy: muscle

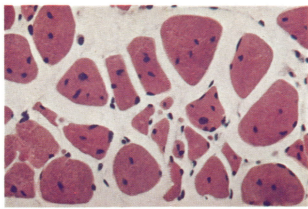

13.62 Muscular dystrophy: muscle

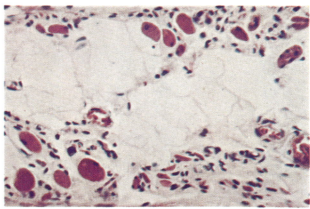

13.63 Muscular dystrophy: muscle

13.55 and **13.56 Rheumatoid arthritis: muscle.** In this disease there is focal interstitial myositis. **13.55** A lymphoid follicle has formed in the interstitial tissues: a 'lymphorrhage'. Similar infiltrates are seen in myasthenia gravis and thyrotoxicosis but not usually in the muscular dystrophies. **13.56** Lymphocytic and plasma cells infiltrate the interstitial tissues round several fibres. One of the fibrils (centre) has undergone floccular degeneration and is being digested by macrophages. **13.57** and **13.58 Dermatomyositis: muscle. 13.57** The fibre in the centre has undergone floccular degeneration and is being phagocytosed. Phagocytosis of degenerating muscle is more characteristic of myositis than of muscular dystrophy. Several other fibres are atrophic and the sarcolemmal nuclei are increased in number. This may be a sign of regeneration. **13.58** The fibres are shrunken and atrophied to varying degrees. Several show central vacuolation, a change that is virtually pathognomonic of polymyositis. **13.59** and **13.60 Neurogenic atrophy: muscle. 13.59** Intact fibres (right) and denervated atrophic fibres (left) lie side by side. The atrophic fibres are very narrow and the number of sarcolemmal nuclei appears to be greatly increased though there is probably no absolute increase in their number. **13.60** This shows several atrophic denervated fibres. The sarcoplasm at the periphery of each is spongy and loose-textured with loss of myofibrils, but the myofibrils in the centre of the fibril still retain their striations. The sarcolemmal nuclei are prominent and appear more numerous than normal because of the shrinkage of the fibres. **13.61 Myotonic dystrophy: muscle.** There has been migration of the muscle nuclei from the periphery of the fibre inwards towards its centre. **13.62** and **13.63 Muscular dystrophy: muscle. 13.62** Migration of the sarcolemmal nuclei into the substance of the fibres is best seen, as here, when the fibres are cut in cross-section. Some of the fibrils are atrophic. Inward migration of nuclei, particularly when widespread, is suggestive of muscular dystrophy and especially myotonic dystrophy. **13.63** There is extensive fatty infiltration and fibrous tissue formation between the atrophic muscle fibres. This change occurs early in muscular dystrophy.

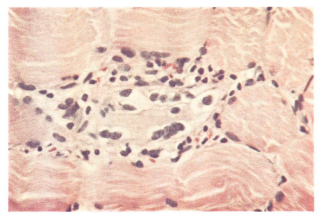

13.64 Muscular dystrophy: muscle

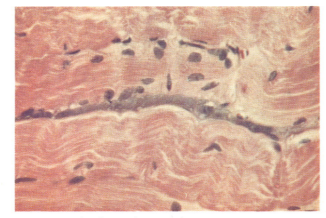

13.65 Muscular dystrophy: muscle

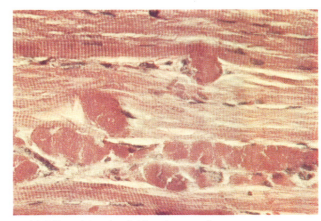

13.66 Idiopathic myoglobinuria: muscle

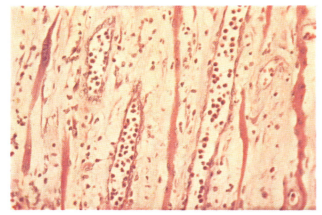

13.67 X-irradiation: muscle

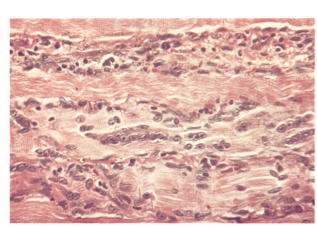

13.68 Anterior tibial compartment syndrome: muscle

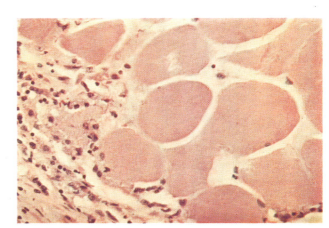

13.69 Infarct: muscle

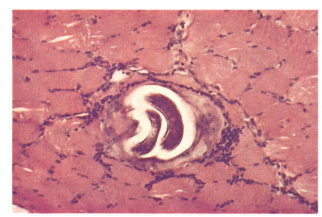

13.70 Trichiniasis: muscle

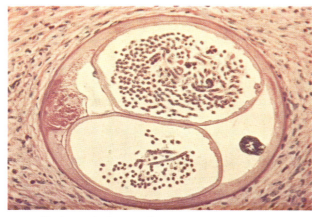

13.71 Onchocerciasis: muscle

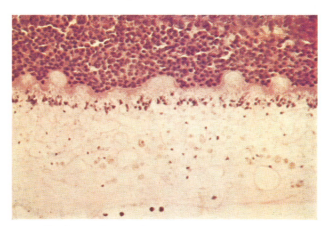

13.72 Cysticercosis: muscle

13.64 and **13.65 Muscular dystrophy: muscle. 13.64** One or more fibres in the centre have completely lost their myofibrils and are represented by a cluster of swollen sarcolemmal nuclei and a little faintly basophilic cytoplasm. **13.65** In the centre is a basophilic fibril. It has lost its myofibrils and consists of basophilic cytoplasm and swollen vesicular sarcolemmal nuclei. **13.66 Idiopathic myoglobinuria: muscle.** The patient, a boy of 5, suffered from sudden attacks of weakness and muscle pain, sometimes after excessive exercise, and then passed dark-coloured urine containing myoglobin. The condition is relatively benign but as in the crush syndrome, death may occur from renal failure. This muscle biopsy shows floccular degeneration and necrosis of several fibres of the peroneus longus. **13.67 X-irradiation: muscle.** Skeletal muscle is fairly radioresistant but here the muscle fibres are shrunken and have lost their striations. The gaps between the fibres are filled with loose connective tissue. The capillaries are greatly dilated and contain many polymorphs. **13.68 Anterior tibial compartment syndrome: muscle.** The lesion is probably the result of haemorrhage and oedema in a rigidly confined space and consequent pressure ischaemia of the muscle. Many of the muscle fibres have degenerated and the large numbers of swollen sarcolemmal nuclei, some in mitosis, are probably evidence of regeneration. Nevertheless there is a marked tendency in this condition to fibrous replacement of the muscle. **13.69 Infarct: muscle.** The muscle is the gastrocnemius. The fibres are swollen, non-striated and lacking nuclei. Macrophages (left) are digesting these necrotic fibres and fibrosis is occurring. **13.70 Trichiniasis: muscle.** This shows an encysted larva of *Trichinella spiralis* in striated muscle. The pale-staining capsule is formed by muscle cells. The neighbouring fibres are compressed and the interstitial tissue is infiltrated by chronic inflammatory cells. Larvae may remain alive for years in this state and infection takes place when raw or partly cooked pork containing larvae is eaten. **13.71 Onchocerciasis: muscle.** This shows an adult female *Onchocerca volvulus* full of embryos. Though enclosed in a dense fibrous nodule the parasite appears to be fully viable. Most fibrous nodules of this type occur in the subcutaneous tissues. **13.72 Cysticercosis: muscle.** This shows the smoothly convoluted surface of the cystic larval form of the worm (*Cysticercus cellulosae*) which was lying among the muscle fibres. A pus-like exudate (top) surrounds the cyst. An acute inflammatory reaction like this usually occurs only when the larva dies. The adult tapeworm *Taenia solium* lives in the small intestine of man. Cysticerci can form in any organ and produce serious lesions.

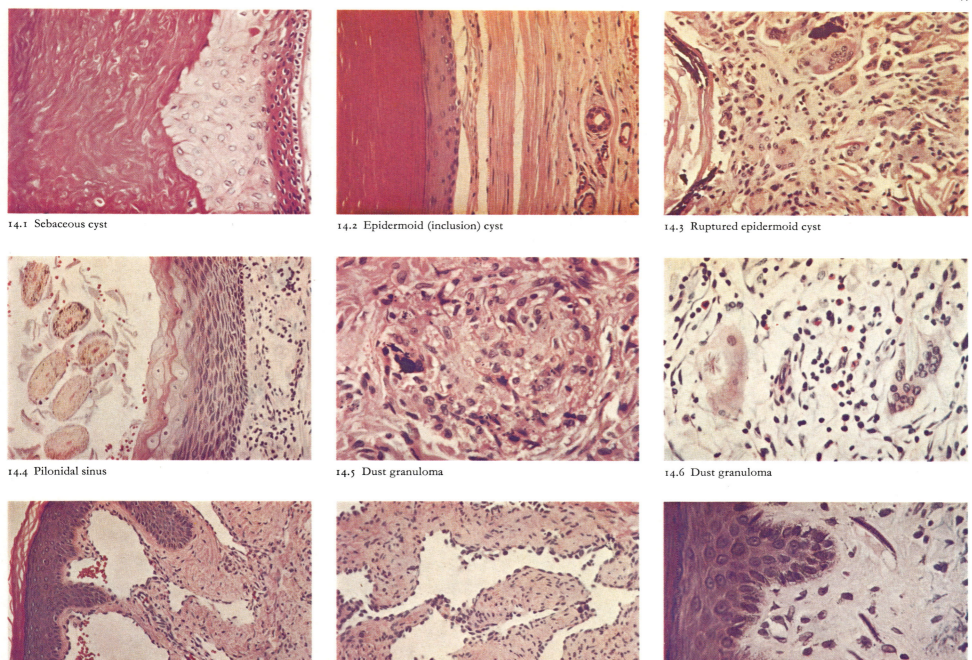

14.1 Sebaceous cyst   14.2 Epidermoid (inclusion) cyst   14.3 Ruptured epidermoid cyst

14.4 Pilonidal sinus   14.5 Dust granuloma   14.6 Dust granuloma

14.7 Capillary haemangioma   14.8 Chronic lymphoedema   14.9 Onchocerciasis

14.1 and 14.2 'Sebaceous' cysts. 14.1 This is a true sebaceous cyst, lined by sebaceous epithelium. **14.2** On the other hand this is an epidermoid (inclusion) cyst, formed by traumatic displacement of epidermis into the deeper layers of the skin. The sweat gland (right) is a skin appendage and not related to the cyst. **14.3 Ruptured epidermoid cyst.** The cyst has ruptured and released keratin and sebaceous material which have excited a granulomatous reaction with numerous macrophages and multinucleate giant cells. Some of the keratin has calcified (dark blue). **14.4 Pilonidal sinus.** This is a section through part of the wall of the sinus which was located in the sacral region. The sinus is lined by epidermis and the lumen (left) contains many hairs and keratinous debris. In the deeper part of the sinus the epithelial lining had broken down and the hairs, desquamated cells and bacteria had excited an acute inflammatory reaction. **14.5 and 14.6 Dust granuloma. 14.5** The patient had been involved in an accident many years previously in which road dust was driven into his skin. Shortly before the biopsy was taken there was a sudden flare-up and numerous nodules formed in the affected part of the skin. This

shows one of the many follicular collections of histiocytes of which the nodules are composed. The cells are of the epithelioid type and the lesion resembles sarcoid. Some of the cells contain black dust particles and the others were shown to contain abundant birefringent material. An altered immune response was probably responsible for the sudden flare-up. **14.6** This is a case similar to 14.5. Crystalline foreign material is present within a multinucleated giant cell (right) and in the other giant cell (left) there is a stellate asteroid body of a type occasionally seen in sarcoidosis. **14.7 Capillary haemangioma.** It consists of large distended capillary-type vessels which extend high into the dermal papillae. **14.8 Chronic lymphoedema.** This is the subcutaneous tissue of the dorsum of the foot. The normal fatty tissues have been replaced by fibrous connective tissue and dilated lymphatic vessels lined by plump endothelial cells. **14.9 Onchocerciasis.** This is the skin adjacent to a subcutaneous Onchocercal nodule that contained adult worms. Several microfilariae (*Onchocerca volvulus*) are present in the dermis but there is no apparent response on the part of the host.

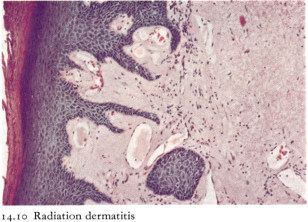

14.10 Radiation dermatitis

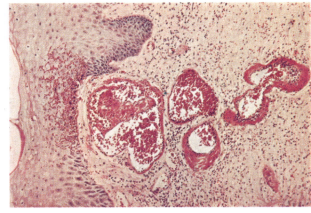

14.11 Radiation dermatitis

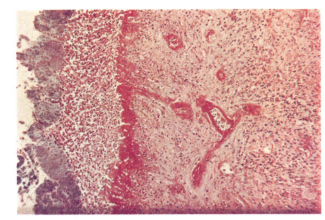

14.12 Radiation dermatitis

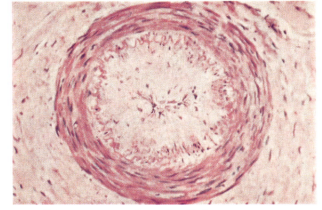

14.13 Cutaneous artery after x-irradiation

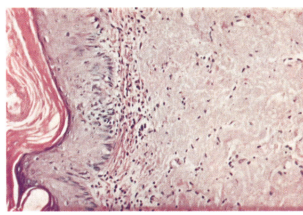

14.14 Senile elastosis

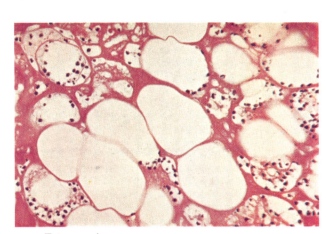

14.15 Fat necrosis

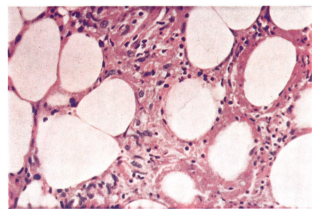

14.16 Fat necrosis

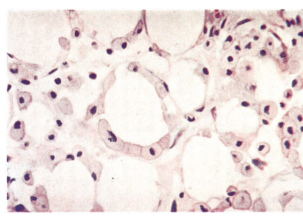

14.17 Fat necrosis

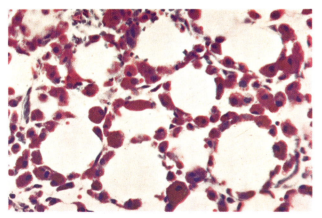

14.18 Fat necrosis

14.10–14.12 Radiation dermatitis. The patient had received therapeutic x-irradiation to the arm 6 months previously. **14.10** The epidermis is hyperplastic and hyperkeratinised (left) with irregular proliferation of the rete ridges. The blood vessels and lymphatics are very dilated. The dermal connective tissue has lost its normal fibrillary structure and is hyaline. **14.11** The blood vessels which have been severely damaged are greatly dilated and fibrinous exudate forms a cuff round them. The epidermal cells are being separated by oedema and haemorrhage. They are dying prematurely and failing to keratinise. These changes lead to ulceration. **14.12** In this region the skin has ulcerated. Colonies of bacteria are growing on the surface (left), and beneath them is an exudate of polymorphs and fibrin. Fibrin also forms a cuff round the blood vessel (right) and there is considerable fibrosis. **14.13 Cutaneous artery after x-irradiation.** The media shows loss of muscle cell nuclei. The internal elastic lamina stains poorly and is broken in places. Abundant poorly cellular connective tissue has formed in the intima and the lumen is almost obliterated. **14.14 Senile elastosis.** The change affects only light-exposed areas and causes the skin to become less elastic than normal. Here the normal fibrous appearance of the subpapillary connective tissue has been replaced by clumped material which stains like elastic tissue and is

thought to contain altered elastic tissue. **14.15–14.18 Fat necrosis. 14.15** This is subcutaneous fat of skin that had received therapeutic radiation. The fat cells have died and each cell has lost its nucleus. The large lipid droplets thus exposed are being attacked and broken down by neutrophil leucocytes (polymorphs). There is also an extensive fibrinous exudate. Dead fat often provokes a prolonged subacute or chronic inflammatory reaction and fibrosis may be considerable. **14.16** In this area some of the fat cells have died but some are still viable. The living cells (left and top) have an intact and well-demarcated boundary whereas the dead fat cells (right) have an indistinct margin and are surrounded by eosinophilic exudate. The lipid within the dead cells is being removed by polymorphs and macrophages and fibrous tissue is forming. **14.17** All the fat cells have died and the large droplet of lipid in each cell's cytoplasm has consequently been exposed to attack by macrophages. The ingested lipid gives the cytoplasm of these macrophages a 'foamy' or 'frosted-glass' appearance. One appears to be in mitosis (left of centre). **14.18** This is a frozen section of the lesion shown in 14.17. The fat has been stained with Sudan IV. The large lipid droplet lying free in the centre of each dead fat cell has dissolved in the staining solution, whereas the lipid inside the macrophages has remained and taken up the dye.

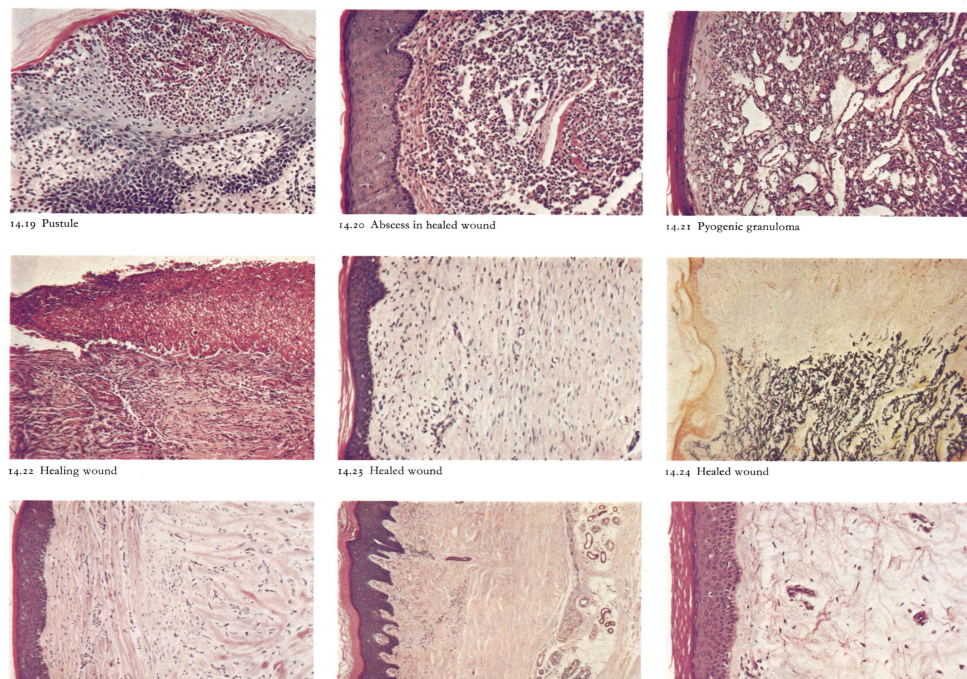

14.19 Pustule

14.20 Abscess in healed wound

14.21 Pyogenic granuloma

14.22 Healing wound

14.23 Healed wound

14.24 Healed wound

14.25 Keloid

14.26 Scleroderma

14.27 Pretibial myxoedema

14.19 Pustule. This is a small pus-filled vesicle lying in the upper layer of the epidermis. Keratin strands mingle with the pus cells. **14.20 Abscess in healed wound.** This is a surgical incision, three weeks old. The epithelium has healed but a small collection of pus has formed in the wound. Suture material and keratin squames mingle with the pus cells. **14.21 Pyogenic granuloma.** The lesion is a polypoid mass of proliferating capillaries and chronic inflammatory cells covered with squamous epithelium. Sometimes the surface ulcerates. **14.22 Healing wound.** The surface is covered by a dense scab of fibrin (above) in which leucocytes are trapped. A sheet of squamous epithelial cells is growing (from the left) beneath the scab across the layer of newly formed vascular connective tissue (below). The scab is loosening and will soon fall off. Epithelial cells can grow only on living tissue and so undermine the scab. **14.23 and 14.24 Healed wound. 14.23** This is the scar of a healed non-infected surgical wound some months old. It consists of mature but still fairly vascular collagenous fibrous tissue. The collagen fibres do not have the interwoven appearance of the normal dermis but are arranged mainly in the horizontal

plane. **14.24** This is a healed surgical incision similar to 14.23. The section, which has been stained to show elastic fibrils, has been taken at the junction between the normal tissue (below) and the scar (above). Elastic fibres are abundant in the normal tissues but completely absent in the scar tissue. **14.25 Keloid.** A keloid is a hypertrophic scar (right) and characteristically consists of thick eosinophilic bands of collagen and large fibroblasts. **14.26 Scleroderma.** The papillary layer of the dermis (left) is normal but beneath it all the collagen of the deeper layers is swollen and hyalinised. This collagen appears relatively acellular but in fact the connective tissue cells are present in normal numbers. They are more widely spaced because of the swelling of the collagen. There is no fibroblastic proliferation or fibrosis involved in this lesion, in contrast to keloid and scar formation. The sweat glands (right) are unaffected. **14.27 Pretibial myxoedema.** This localised lesion is associated with thyrotoxicosis. The vessels, cells and connective tissue fibrils are widely separated by large amounts of hydrophilic ground-substance which fails to stain. The ground-substance is largely mucopolysaccharide in nature.

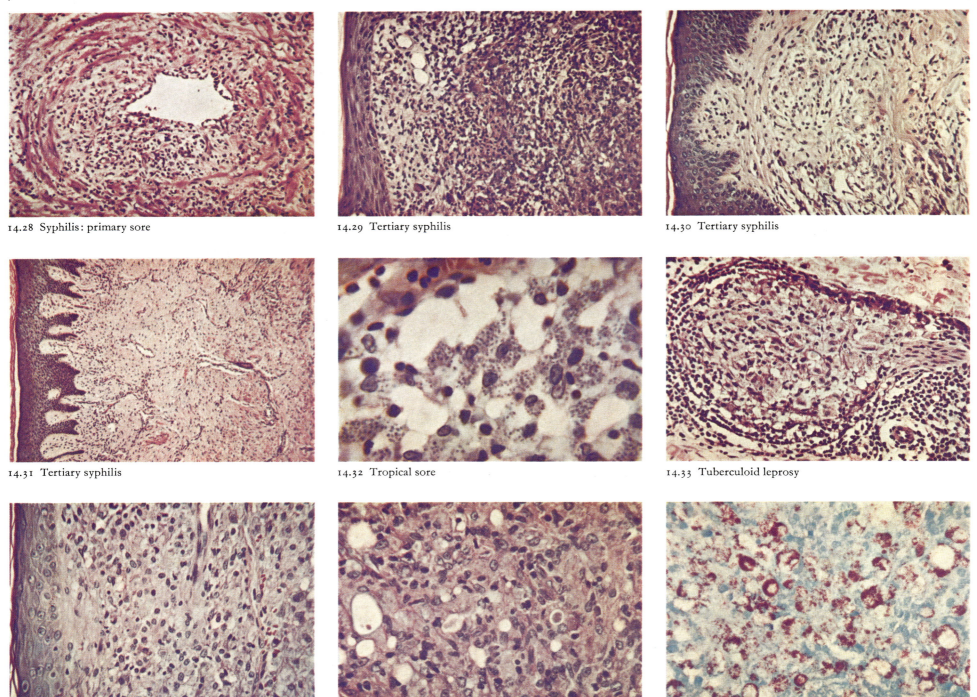

14.28 Syphilis: primary sore

14.29 Tertiary syphilis

14.30 Tertiary syphilis

14.31 Tertiary syphilis

14.32 Tropical sore

14.33 Tuberculoid leprosy

14.34 Lepromatous (nodular) leprosy

14.35 Lepromatous leprosy

14.36 Lepromatous leprosy

14.28 Syphilis: primary sore. There is very pronounced endophlebitis in this small venule, and plasma cells and lymphocytes are present in all coats of the vessel but are particularly numerous in the thickened intima. The lumen is greatly reduced. When many vessels are affected in this way, and especially when thrombosis occurs to occlude them completely, necrosis and ulceration result. **14.29–14.31 Tertiary syphilis. 14.29** This is an early active lesion. There is an intense granulomatous reaction in the dermis. The exudate is rich in macrophages (some multinucleate), lymphocytes, plasma cells and fibroblasts. These inflammatory lesions are often highly destructive especially when accompanied as they usually are by obliterative endarteritis. Consequently fibrosis is a feature of more chronic lesions. **14.30** This is a more advanced lesion than 14.29. A central necrotic focus is surrounded by macrophages, with lymphocytes and plasma cells at the periphery. Early fibrosis is evident in and around the lesion. **14.31** This is a late stage. Most of the inflammatory reaction shown in 14.29 and 14.30 has disappeared and the skin is left heavily and uniformly fibrosed. **14.32 Tropical sore.** The lesion is a tuberculoid granuloma which consists of swollen histiocytes which have in their cytoplasm large numbers of the

causative organism, *Leishmania tropicani.* **14.33 Tuberculoid leprosy.** A tuberculoid fucos has formed in a small nerve in the subcutaneous tissues. Lymphocytes form a cuff round the lesion. A small part of the nerve is visible on the right. In this type of lesion acid-fast bacilli are not likely to be found. **14.34–14.36 Lepromatous (nodular) leprosy. 14.34** Except for a narrow zone beneath the epidermis (left), the dermis is packed with macrophages (lepra cells) which have distinct cell boundaries and which do not form follicles. A few lymphocytes are present. **14.35** This is at a slightly higher magnification, to show the characteristic vacuoles within some of the macrophages (Virchow cells). Some of the vacuoles appear empty probably because the contents have been lost during processing. Other vacuoles contain dense clumps of leprosy bacilli (right of centre, for example). **14.36** This is the same lesion as 14.35 stained by the Fite Faraco method to show the large numbers of acid-fast leprosy bacilli (stained magenta) within the lepra cells. In some cells the bacilli are scattered throughout the cytoplasm, in others they are aggregated into clumps within vacuoles.

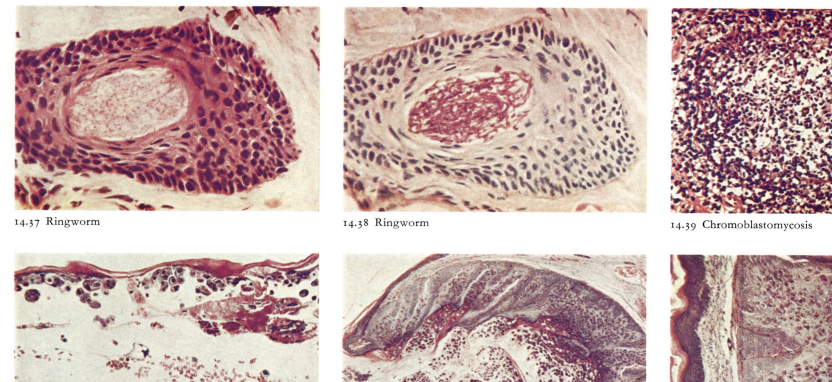
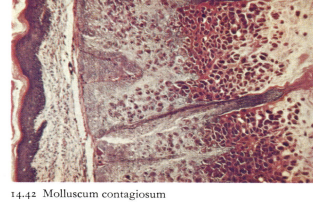

14.37 Ringworm   14.38 Ringworm   14.39 Chromoblastomycosis

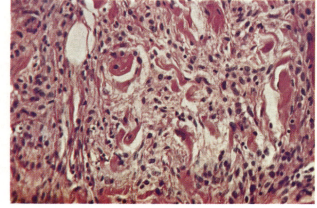
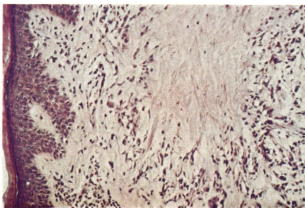
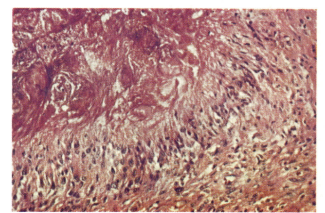

14.40 Varicella (chicken pox)   14.41 Molluscum contagiosum   14.42 Molluscum contagiosum

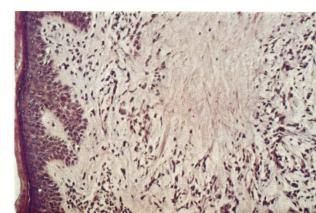

14.43 Granuloma annulare   14.44 Granuloma annulare   14.45 Rheumatoid nodule

14.37 and **14.38 Ringworm. 14.37** This is a section of a hair follicle. The keratin of the hair shaft has been destroyed and replaced by a compact mass of filaments of *Microsporon audouini* (centre). **14.38** This is the same lesion as 14.37. Here the section has been subjected to the periodic acid-Schiff method which stains the filamentous organism magenta. **14.39 Chromoblastomycosis.** The patient had a large chronic ulcer on the dorsum of his foot. This shows one of the small abscesses that were present in large numbers in the subcutaneous tissues. Within it a cluster of the characteristic dark-brown oval organisms can be seen, as well as single organisms The cellular infiltrate consists of polymorphs, lymphocytes, macrophages and fibroblasts. **14.40 Varicella (chicken pox).** The lesion is an intra-epidermal bulla which forms as a result of degeneration of the epithelial cells. Rounded-up swollen cells have been desquamated into the lumen. These are the 'balloon' cells obtained on aspiration. **14.41** and **14.42 Molluscum contagiosum.** This lesion is virus-induced and usually multiple. **14.41** The characteristic flask shape of the nodule is evident. **14.42** The prickle cells of the epidermis are enlarged and their cytoplasm contains homogeneous eosinophilic structures (molluscum bodies) which are aggregations

of elementary bodies. The cell nuclei are flat and inconspicuous. **14.43** and **14.44 Granuloma annulare. 14.43** This is an early necrobiotic focus. The thick collagen bundles of the dermis are becoming broken up and separated by histiocytes and fibroblasts proliferating between them. **14.44** A fairly large focus of necrotic collagen is present (above) in the dermis, surrounded by histiocytes that show a slight tendency to palisading. Palisading is often a more marked feature than here and then the lesion more closely resembles the rheumatoid nodule, particularly since mucinous material is present in both. However the superficial position of the lesion contrasts with the subcutaneous site of the rheumatoid nodule. Distinction from necrobiosis lipoidica may be more difficult. Helpful features are the absence of lipid, giant cells, vascular changes and epidermal atrophy. **14.45 Rheumatoid nodule.** The centre of the nodule (above left) consists of dead connective tissue which still shows its fibrillary composition, in contrast to the more amorphous necrotic material found in granulomatous lesions such as tuberculosis. The necrotic tissue stains a deep red (fibrinoid) and it is enclosed by histiocytes which typically show well-developed palisading of the nuclei.

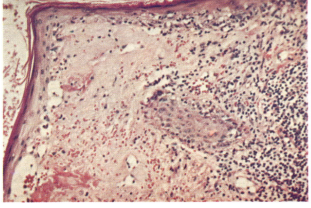

14.46 Acute lupus erythematosus

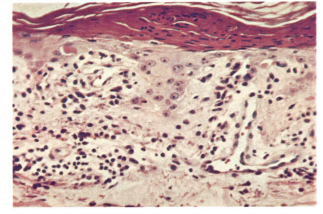

14.47 Lupus erythematosus

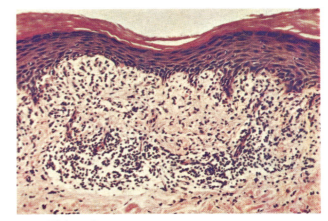

14.48 Lichen planus

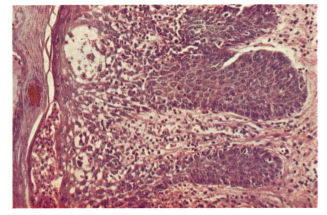

14.49 Eczema

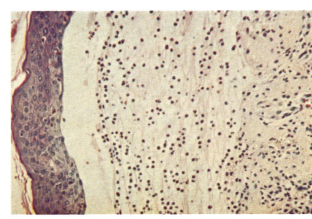

14.50 Dermatitis herpetiformis

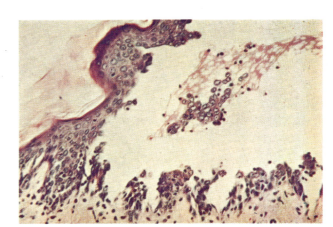

14.51 Pemphigus vulgaris

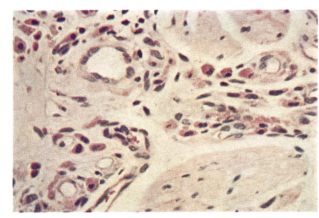

14.52 Urticaria pigmentosa

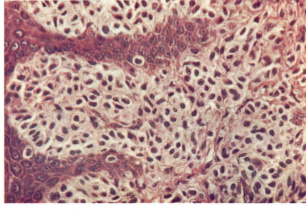

14.53 Mast cell naevus

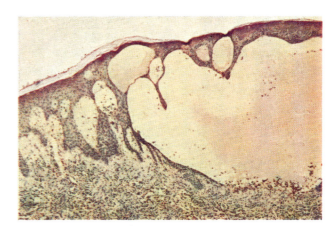

14.54 Erythema multiforme

14.46 Acute lupus erythematosus. The epidermis is atrophic and the basal layer shows severe liquefaction degeneration. The subepithelial tissues are extremely oedematous and hyaline and there are deposits of fibrin. A band of lymphocytic infiltration is present (right) beneath the damaged part of the dermis. **14.47 Lupus erythematosus.** The changes mainly affect the epithelium which, though extremely atrophic, is hyperkeratinised. Much of the keratin is nucleated (parakeratosis). The basal layer is almost destroyed by liquefaction degeneration. The papillary layer of the dermis is oedematous and contains a few lymphocytes. Pigment has been lost from the cells of the basal layers and taken up by histiocytes. **14.48 Lichen planus.** There is hyperkeratosis and the stratum granulosum is prominent. The rete ridges are saw-toothed. Often they are also lengthened. There is an infiltrate of lymphocytes and macrophages that goes right up to the epidermis but is sharply limited to the papillary and subpapillary layers of the dermis. The basal cell layer is present. Sometimes it is destroyed. **14.49 Eczema.** The main features are oedema within the epithelium (spongiosis) and disintegration of clumps of epithelial cells, with the formation of vesicles. Three successive stages of vesicle formation are seen here, the latest lesion (bottom left) being full of polymorphs (pustule formation). The papillae are oedematous and their vessels distended. The rete ridges are correspondingly elongated. **14.50 Dermatitis herpetiformis.** The entire epidermis has separated from the dermis to form a large vesicle

(centre) containing numerous polymorphs, some of which are eosinophils, and a few strands of fibrin. The dermis is infiltrated with inflammatory cells. **14.51 Pemphigus vulgaris.** This shows one end of a bulla. It is suprabasal in position and has been formed by loss of cohesion between the cells of the lower malpighian layers of the epidermis (acantholysis). The roof and floor appear ragged where epithelial cells are becoming detached and falling into the lumen, where they float singly or in clusters. **14.52 Urticaria pigmentosa.** In this condition the main abnormality is an excessive number of mast cells round the small dermal blood vessels. Though in this section the mast cell cytoplasm is intensely eosinophilic, it is sometimes basophilic. **14.53 Mast cell naevus.** The lesion is a nodule formed of densely-packed mast cells. The cells possess abundant granular cytoplasm and have a distinct cell border. The rete ridges are elongated and the clear cells within the basal epithelium are melanocytes. **14.54 Erythema multiforme.** The bulla is subepidermal at its centre (right) but intra-epidermal at the periphery (centre). There are also intra-epidermal 'spongiotic' vesicles and the dermis is heavily infiltrated with acute and chronic inflammatory cells. A similar histological picture of bulla formation may be seen in bullous pemphigoid and in dermatitis herpetiformis but in these lesions the number of eosinophil polymorphs in the bulla and in the dermis tends to be large.

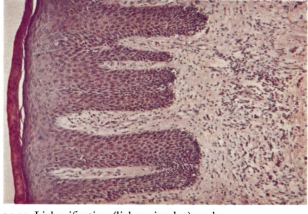

14.55 Lichenification (lichen simplex): vulva

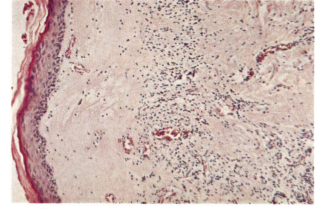

14.56 Lichen sclerosis: vulva

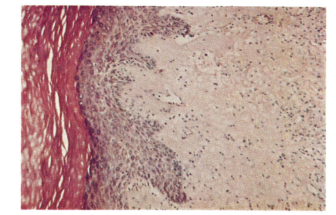

14.57 Leukoplakia: vulva

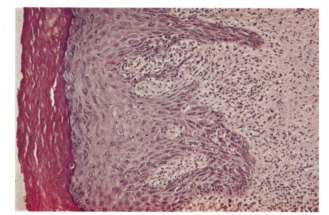

14.58 Leukoplakia: vulva

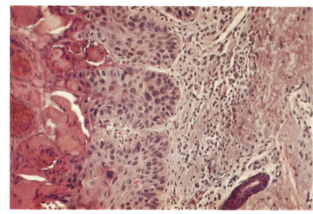

14.59 Senile keratosis

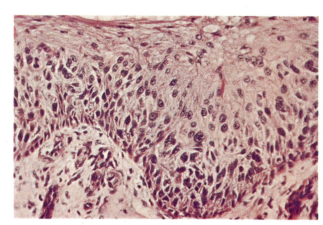

14.60 Bowen's disease

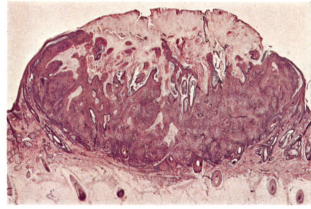

14.61 Kerato-acanthoma (molluscum sebaceum)

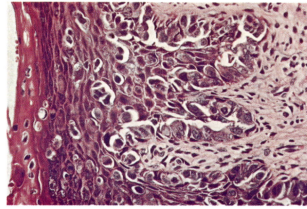

14.62 Paget's disease of nipple

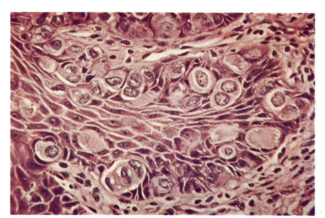

14.63 Extramammary Paget's disease

14.55–14.58 are at the same magnification, to allow comparison. **14.55 Lichenification (lichen simplex): vulva.** This lesion is a reaction to chronic irritation such as scratching and is fully reversible. The papillae are greatly elongated and the rete ridges are correspondingly longer. The epithelial hyperplasia is of a selective nature, affecting only the papillae and not the intervening surface epithelium. There is disorganisation of keratin formation with persistence of nuclei (parakeratosis). A chronic inflammatory cellular exudate is present in the underlying tissues. **14.56 Lichen sclerosis: vulva.** The epithelium is flat and atrophic, and the papillae are inconspicuous. Keratin is present in excess but it is not nucleated. The most noteworthy feature is the hyalinisation, perhaps from oedema of the collagenous tissue beneath the epithelium. This is separated from the deeper layers by a sharply defined band of chronic inflammatory cells. **14.57 and 14.58 Leukoplakia: vulva. 14.57** There is evidence of lichen sclerosis, in the form of hyalinisation of the subepithelial tissues. However the epithelium is more heavily keratinised than 14.56; and in contrast to 14.55, it shows overall hyperplasia, the pattern being unlike that of normal epithelium. **14.58** The features are the same as 14.57 but the lesion is a more advanced one. The number of chronic inflammatory cells is considerably greater. **14.59 Senile keratosis.** There is hyperkeratosis and the cells of the malpighian layer show irregular downward proliferation, as well as a disorderly arrangement. There is an infiltrate of chronic inflammatory cells in the upper dermis. There is also marked elastosis (solar degeneration) (right) and

exposure to the sun is an important aetiological factor in this precancerous condition. **14.60 Bowen's disease.** The lesion is a non-invasive squamous cell carcinoma. The whole structure of the epithelium and its layering is disorganised; and the epithelial cells show great variation in size, shape and nuclear structure. **14.61 Kerato-acanthoma (molluscum sebaceum).** This lesion grows rapidly for 2–3 months and then regresses, so that the whole life cycle occupies less than 6 months. It is confined to hair-bearing skin and has its origin in pilosebaceous follicles. It consists of a craterlike structure whose floor is formed of intensely hyperplastic epithelium with an inflammatory margin. **14.62 Paget's disease of nipple.** Large atypical cells with slightly basophilic cytoplasm (Paget's cells) are present in large numbers in the basal layers of the epithelium and in smaller numbers in the other layers. These cells although lying in intimate relationship with the squamous epithelium do not form an integral part of the epithelium, whose cells are displaced and have undergone pressure atrophy but show no signs of being tumorous, in contrast to Bowen's disease. The presence of Paget's disease in the nipple signifies the presence of a carcinoma in the underlying breast. **14.63 Extramammary Paget's disease.** This lesion was in the anal canal and being at a higher power view than 14.62 it shows the differences between the Paget's cells and the squamous epithelial cells, and how one has been displaced and deformed by the other.

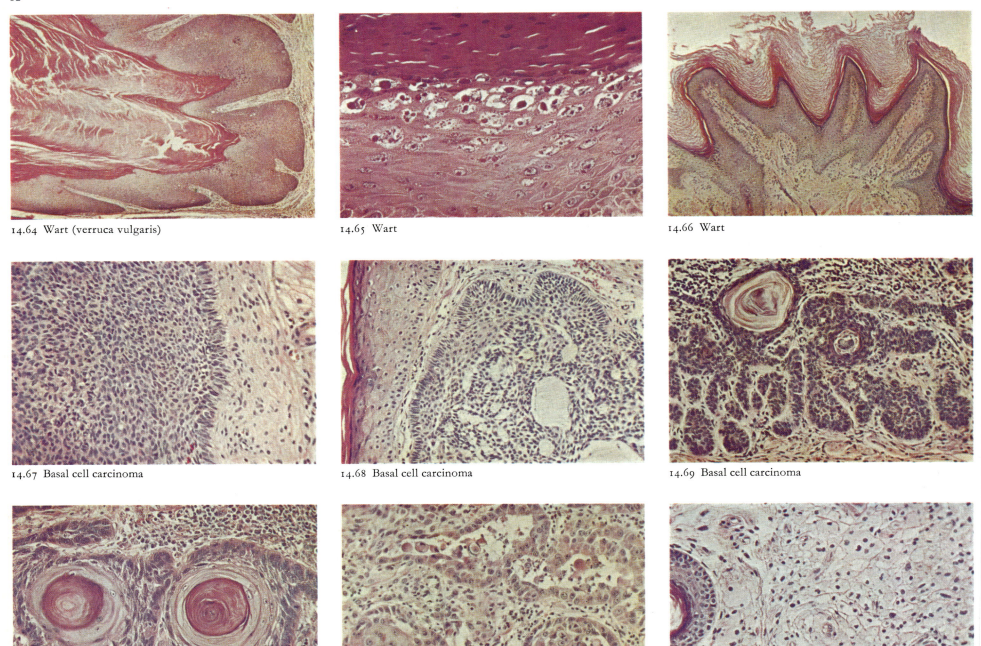

14.64 Wart (verruca vulgaris)

14.65 Wart

14.66 Wart

14.67 Basal cell carcinoma

14.68 Basal cell carcinoma

14.69 Basal cell carcinoma

14.70 Squamous cell carcinoma

14.71 Squamous cell carcinoma

14.72 Xanthelasma

14.64–14.66 Wart (verruca vulgaris). 14.64 The epidermis is hyperplastic, forming a bulbous crypt (left) from which massive quantities of keratin (left) have been produced. At this magnification the granular layer is obviously overdeveloped. **14.65** This is a high-power view of the outer layers of the epidermis in an active virus wart. As the epithelial cells move outwards to form the granular layer, many of them, as a result of viral damage, become vacuolated and instead of forming normal keratohyalin granules develop large deeply eosinophilic masses within their cytoplasm. The keratin produced by the epithelial cells in this damaged condition is often nucleated (parakeratosis). True virus inclusions are not visible in ordinary preparations. **14.66** This lesion represents a virus wart in which viral damage to the epithelium has ceased to be evident. The skin is left with an abnormal papillary architecture. **14.67–14.69 Basal cell carcinoma. 14.67** This is the advancing edge of the tumour. It consists of a large solid mass of tumour cells which are small, close-packed and basophilic. In this example there is no differentiation into prickle cells. The peripheral cells are columnar and palisaded. **14.68** In this example the epithelial masses are becoming oedematous and breaking down to form small cystic spaces filled with watery secretion. Some of the cells in the central part of the mass have differentiated into prickle cells but around the margin they are palisaded and typically basal cell in appearance. **14.69** In this lesion the epithelial masses are much smaller but like the others are composed of small close-packed basal-type cells. In the centre of two of the masses the cells are differentiating into keratin. The transition from basal cells to keratin is abrupt. Lymphocytes are present. In basal cell carcinomas the peripheral cells are always basophilic basal cell types, even though the central cells are keratinising, whereas in squamous cell carcinomas the peripheral cells are large eosinophilic prickle cells. **14.70 and 14.71 Squamous cell carcinoma. 14.70** This shows two 'cell nests' or epithelial 'pearls'. Each consists of a central laminated mass of keratin surrounded by flattened squamous cells which are in turn enclosed within prickle cells. **14.71** This tumour is unusual in its tendency to form a 'pseudoglandular' structure. **14.72 Xanthelasma.** The lesion was a yellow plaque situated at the inner canthus. The upper dermis is full of discrete lipid-laden macrophages, some multinucleate.

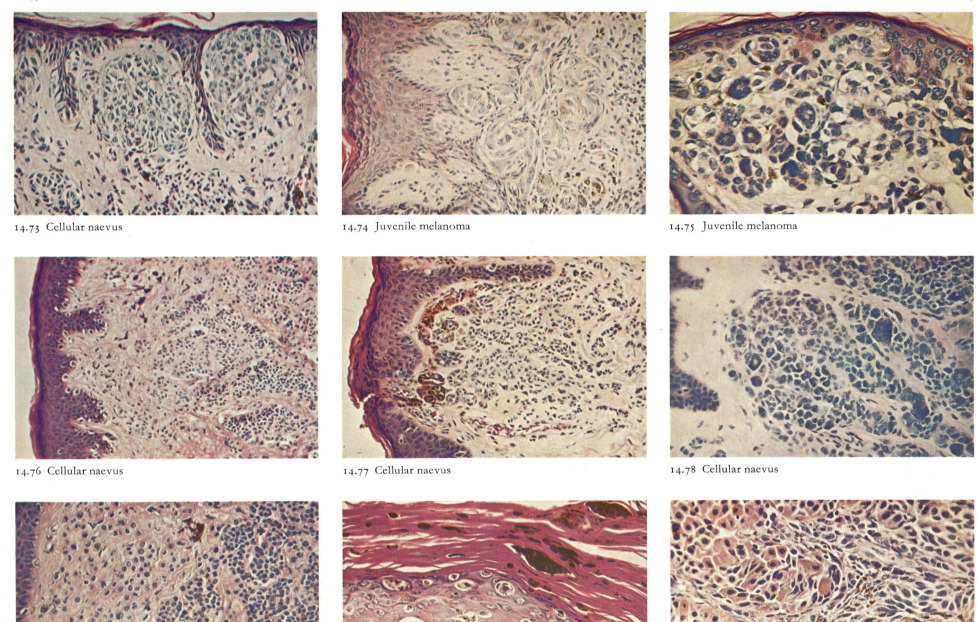

14.73 Cellular naevus

14.74 Juvenile melanoma

14.75 Juvenile melanoma

14.76 Cellular naevus

14.77 Cellular naevus

14.78 Cellular naevus

14.79 Cellular naevus

14.80 Malignant melanoma

14.81 Malignant melanoma

14.73 Cellular naevus. This is a cellular naevus from a child. There is proliferation of melanocytes within the basal layer of the epithelium leading to the production of nests of these cells which as they become larger are extruded into the underlying connective tissue. At this stage most of the melanocytes contain pigment but later melanogenesis would cease in most of them. **14.74** and **14.75 Juvenile melanoma.** This is a lesion which arises and grows rapidly in young children and although it often has an alarmingly malignant-looking histology, it is benign and self-limiting. Malignant melanomas are rare before puberty and a tumour may appear malignant yet fail to metastasize. **14.74** This section shows one in an active stage of formation with nests of atypical melanocytes within the lower margin of the hyperplastic epithelium. Some of the abnormal melanocytes have 'invaded' the underlying connective tissue. **14.75** In this specimen, which occurred in a 12-year-old boy, the tumour cells are large and the nuclei are very basophilic. Some of the cells are multinucleate and many are vacuolated. The dermis is oedematous. There was no recurrence after resection. **14.76–14.79 Cellular naevus. 14.76** This is an adult lesion undergoing involutionary changes. The nests of melanocytes (naevus cells) within the dermis are becoming less well defined and some have disappeared, leaving only melanin-containing histiocytes. Note that the surface epidermis still contains an excess layer of large melano-

cytes within its basal layer. This is important because it is these abnormal intra-epidermal melanocytes which might at some later date give rise to a malignant melanoma. **14.77** This shows part of an adult lesion in which proliferation of melanocytes has ceased. Those which were previously produced and extruded into the dermis now lie in rounded clumps and cords. Only those nearest the surface continue to form pigment. The overlying epidermis still contains an excess of rather prominent melanocytes within its basal layer (lentigo). The epidermis shows a very small traumatic ulcer. **14.78** The naevus cells, many of which are multinucleate, show regressive changes and their nuclear staining is irregular and 'smudgy' **14.79** Like 14.78 this shows involutionary changes. Note especially the more superficial melanocytes which have rounded up and now resemble cartilage cells. There are relatively few melanocytes in the basal layer of the epidermis. **14.80** and **14.81 Malignant melanoma. 14.80** There is active proliferation of melanocytes within the epidermis and the cells are being shed either singly or as clumps through the upper layers and into the keratin. This is a sign of malignant transformation in a cellular naevus. **14.81** The cells vary greatly in size and shape and range from spindle cells to large epithelioid cells. Their content of melanin varies considerably too, and some, particularly the spindle cells, appear pigment-free.

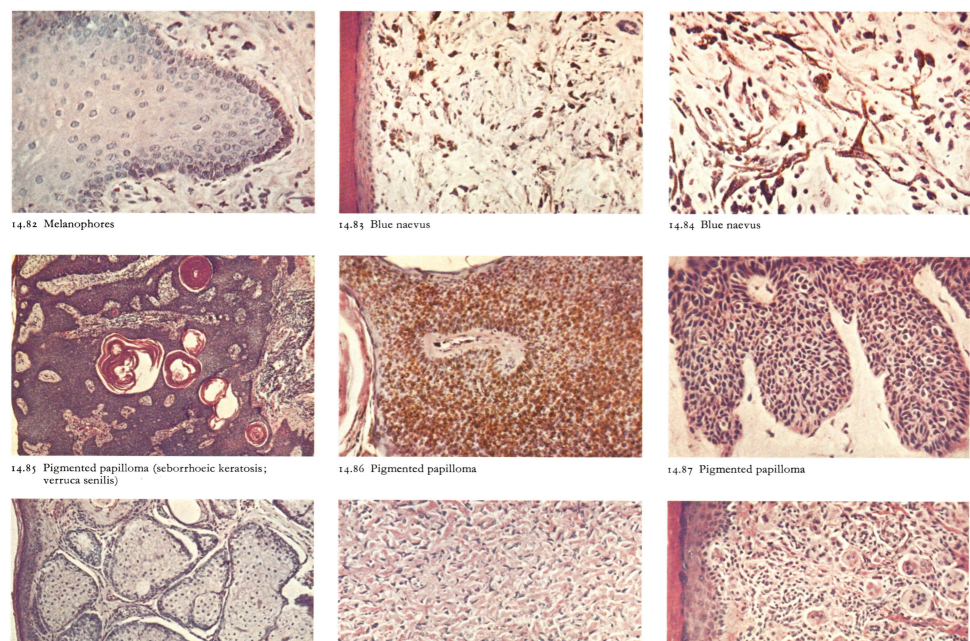

14.82 Melanophores

14.83 Blue naevus

14.84 Blue naevus

14.85 Pigmented papilloma (seborrhoeic keratosis; verruca senilis)

14.86 Pigmented papilloma

14.87 Pigmented papilloma

14.88 Sebaceous gland 'adenoma'

14.89 Dermatofibroma

14.90 Giant-cell reticulohistiocytoma

14.82 Melanophores. The skin shows increased pigmentation. The pigment is concentrated in the basal layers, and in the connective tissue beneath the epithelium there are several histiocytes containing melanin (melanophores). **14.83** and **14.84 Blue naevus. 14.83** The dermis is diffusely infiltrated by melanin-containing cells, many of which are histiocytes (melanophores). The pigment is being produced by spindle-shaped cells with branching processes (dermal melanocytes) which lie in relationship to the dermal collagen bundles. These melanocytes are shown in detail in **14.84**. **14.85–14.87 Pigmented papilloma (seborrhoeic keratosis; verruca senilis). 14.85** The epidermis is greatly thickened and within it are nests of laminated keratin. The cells forming the lesion are prickle cells, though many melanocytes are also present. Melanin pigment is also present but it is not visible at this magnification. **14.86** This is part of one of the epithelial masses. The cells are characteristically small and closely packed, and their cytoplasm contains large quantities of melanin. **14.87** In this field numerous melanocytes stand out as 'clear' cells.

14.88 Sebaceous gland 'adenoma'. The lesion consists of an excessive number of sebaceous glands of an abnormally large size. Apart from its quantitative abnormality the sebaceous tissue appears normal. Sebaceous gland adenomas have an association with tuberous sclerosis. **14.89 Dermatofibroma.** This lesion is well-demarcated but not encapsulated. Stellate and elongated cells of very uniform type lie between intertwining bands of fibrous material. Sometimes many histiocytes are present which contain lipid and/or haemosiderin. The lesion is then a histiocytoma. In some histiocytomas there are also many capillaries and foreign-body giant cells. **14.90 Giant-cell reticulohistiocytoma.** This is a granulomatous lesion and not a neoplasm. It contains many giant cells which are well demarcated and possess finely granular (lipid-rich) cytoplasm. Each giant cell has several vesicular nuclei. The giant cells are embedded in a fibrous stroma.

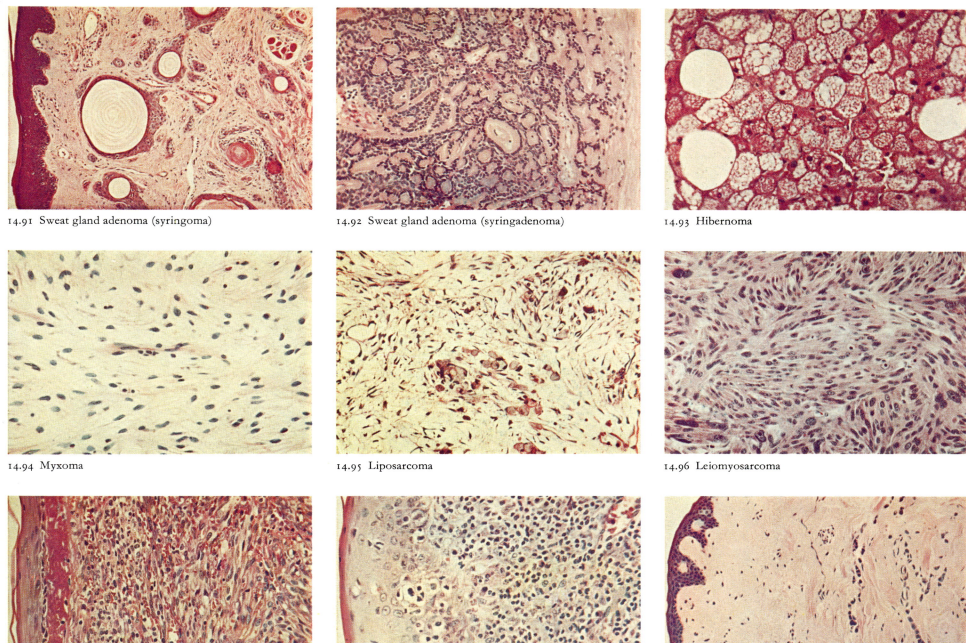

14.91 Sweat gland adenoma (syringoma)

14.92 Sweat gland adenoma (syringadenoma)

14.93 Hibernoma

14.94 Myxoma

14.95 Liposarcoma

14.96 Leiomyosarcoma

14.97 Kaposi's sarcoma

14.98 Mycosis fungoides

14.99 Carcinoma cells in lymphatics

14.91 Sweat gland adenoma (syringoma). These lesions present as multiple small papules, often with irritation, on the chest and abdomen of young adults. Each lesion consists of a collection of tiny tubules and cystic structures formed of keratinising squamous epithelium. These are thought to represent malformed sweat ducts probably of apocrine type. **14.92 Sweat gland adenoma (syringadenoma).** The tumour cells form a reticulum of irregular cords, some of which differentiate into duct-like structures. The epithelial elements are separated by hyaline material. This hyalinised stroma often provides a clue to the sweat-gland origin of a tumour. **14.93 Hibernoma.** Two types of fat cell are present in this tumour of fatty tissue. A few are the large clear cells of normal adult fat, but most are the smaller granular type usually found in the fetus (mulberry cells). This is the type of cell that constitutes brown fat. Brown fat is abundant in hibernating animals: hence the name of the lesion. **14.94 Myxoma.** Macroscopically the tumour was soft and gelatinous. The tumour cells have large nuclei and the cytoplasm is drawn out. They are embedded in a very abundant matrix which contains relatively few collagen fibres but large amounts of poorly-staining ground-substance. **14.95 Liposarcoma.** A frozen section showed abundant fat. The lesion consists mainly of myxosarcomatous tissue composed of stel-

late cells embedded in pale-staining matrix but clusters of young fat cells are visible in the centre. **14.96 Leiomyosarcoma.** The tumour was situated in the scrotum. It consists of interlacing bundles of poorly differentiated smooth muscle cells. The large elongated nuclei of the tumour cells show a remarkable degree of pleomorphism and some are very large. All have prominent nucleoli. There are occasional mitoses (left centre, for example). **14.97 Kaposi's sarcoma.** This is an angiosarcoma. The tumour cells are spindle-shaped and resemble smooth muscle. Mitotic figures are numerous. There is considerable haemorrhage throughout the tumour and particularly beneath the epidermis. **14.98 Mycosis fungoides.** This lesion affects the skin primarily but the viscera may be involved in the later stages. The upper dermis is heavily infiltrated with cells of many varieties, including large cells with deeply-staining and irregularly shaped nuclei (mycosis cells). Note that the cells of the infiltrate are extending up into the interstices of the epithelium to form 'micro-abscesses' of Pautrier. **14.99 Carcinoma cells in lymphatics.** The primary tumour was in breast. Large cells with basophilic, pleomorphic nuclei are lying in the lymphatic channels of the dermis. The skin is oedematous.

INDEX